TALES OF LINDA

ISBN-13: 9781497570849
ISBN-10: 1497570840

The remembrances recorded within were generously supplied by friends, family, colleagues and patients of Dr. Linda Laubenstein. Occasionally changes were made for the sake of clarity or to eliminate a dated reference I apologize for any errors or omissions that may have happened during the transcription and editing process.

I wish to thank everyone who participated in this project.

Priscilla Laubenstein

TALES OF LINDA

Patients, colleagues, friends and family remember

Dr. Linda Laubenstein,
an AIDS pioneer.

CONTENTS

Dr. Edward L. Amorosi: hematology

In Memoriam—61
Flora Davidson: Associate Dean, Barnard College

Patients' Letters:
Rosemarie—64
Bill—65

Linda's Milestones—67

Curriculum Vitae—69

Publications—70

Linda on:

My Family—73

My Friends—75

My Pets—77

School Days—79

Hobbies—81

Vacation Days—82

Sixth Grade—84

DEDICATION

To George, Linda's loving Dad

DESCRIPTION OF A GENUINELY SUCCESSFUL LIFE

"To laugh often and love much;

to win the respect of intelligent persons and the affection of children;

to earn the approbation of honest citizens and endure the betrayal of false friends;

to appreciate beauty; to find the best in others; to give of one's self;

to leave the world a bit better, whether by a healthy child, a garden patch or a redeemed social condition;

to have played and laughed with enthusiasm and sung with exultation;

to know even one life has breathed easier because you have lived—

this is to have succeeded."

Ralph Waldo Emerson

RECOLLECTIONS OF A MOTHER

Priscilla Laubenstein

When our first child was born, we knew almost from the beginning of her life that she was special. She walked soon after she began to crawl and she talked in sentences at an early age. I know that most parents feel the same about their children and maybe with justification, but our judgment was soundly based and confirmed by doctors and friends. From the start, her eyes were dark brown and large, astonishingly large and the one feature that would continue to dominate her face for the rest of her life.

When I look back, I can remember Linda when she was four, playing in the garden and demanding to know the names of flowers. She questioned why some were in bloom and others were not. From an early age she was fascinated by the unknown and continually questioned her father who was working in his vegetable garden. My husband, George, was a patient, loving man. He never failed to answer each and every one of his daughter's questions. Her love of nature and flowers would continue throughout her life. Her constantly questioning and asking why would also continue in adulthood.

I am reminded of Frederick Allen's book Only Yesterday. For me, it seems only yesterday or maybe a lifetime ago, my life was changed and my husband's life was changed. Don't misunderstand. I never wanted anyone to feel sorry for us. We were not the ones who suffered, but our child. Suddenly that little girl in the garden became someone else.

We had put the children to bed. Our second child, Peter, was one and a half, a plump bundle of joy. We sat reading. I can't remember the names of the books, but every now and then George would laugh. He loved to read and he loved working in his vegetable garden and he adored his children. George told me he had purchased a mask for Halloween and he planned to take Linda trick-or-treating. He informed me that I was to stay home with Peter, and that was all right with me. I wanted to tell George how lucky Linda was to have him as a father.

The house was quiet, almost as if an unnatural peace had enveloped us. Then the quiet was broken by a shrill cry. Our first thought was that Linda was playing games, that she was not ready for bed and needed attention—another kiss goodnight, another story, anything that would keep her awake and ready for entertainment. Another scream. George got up from his chair. "I'll see what's going on. That child has the lungs of a little devil." We both moved quickly and entered Linda's bedroom. She had fallen out of bed. She lay crumpled on the floor. "Mom, Dad," she said, "I can't walk. I can't walk." George picked her up and put her back into the bed, "Pris, call the doctor".

I didn't hesitate. The call was made. The doctor assured me that he would come immediately, but it seemed forever before he arrived. "I want to examine the child alone," he said. Reluctantly, we left the room.

"Your daughter has polio. I have seen two other youngsters and they too have polio." Only a few weeks prior, George told me that he had purchased polio insurance for $25. "I think I purchased the insurance so that it would turn out to be a waste of money—insurance against the unthinkable."

"We have another child, doctor," I said. "Would you examine our son?"

"Let me wash my hands. Take your daughter to the Chapin Hospital, a facility for infectious diseases."

George and I were not allowed to accompany our daughter while she was examined. We were not permitted to enter her room. We were told that a spinal tap would be done. Promptly our little five year old was put into an iron lung. The crying had stopped. We worried that Linda would be afraid of the big contraption, that she would think we had deserted her, but she was so accepting because she could now breathe.

I had loved my husband during his courtship. I loved George when we married. But in no way did those emotions compare to the overwhelming love I then felt for my husband. His only concerns were for our daughter and me. Almost at once the gentle man had become a tower of strength. He imparted that strength to me.

Linda was diagnosed with bulbar polio, which affected not only her lungs but her whole body. My father was a physician and my grandfather, also a physician, was one of the founders of Tufts Medical School. I contacted Linda's pediatrician who was associated with Children's Hospital in Boston. Without hesitation, he came to Rhode Island to see Linda. I almost wished he had not come. His diagnosis was grim. He said that Linda had only a short time to live. Neither George nor I wanted to believe him. It was as if we willed our daughter to live. Somehow we knew that our little child was a fighter. Indeed she was a fighter, as a child, as a teenager, as an adult. I shall never know if it was the will to live or divine intervention that tipped the scales.

Within three months, Linda was out of the iron lung. When she was in the hospital, we could not go into her isolation room. We were able to read to her—not the nursery rhymes which she had long grown out of, but stories from the Wonder Books—stories of adventure, danger and the willingness to fight for lost causes.

Thus, our child grew and developed not only in her body, but also in her mind. She spent those early years always questioning. We prayed that we could provide her with the right answers.

I can remember the last words she spoke before entering the hospital. "Dad," she said, "are we going to miss Halloween?" As a child, she didn't have the chance to put on a mask. As an adult, she wore her mask with humor and grace.

I won't say life was easy, but I never thought of myself as a martyr. It was taking one day at a time. I know that's a cliché, but that was the way it was. There was our son Peter who we were determined would not be neglected, although at times it was hard to give our young son the attention he needed, the attention he craved. We were grateful that our two children liked each other. More than that, they loved each other. Had any antagonism appeared, life for our family would have been impossible. I shall always be grateful to Peter for loving his older sister, for his being content to play alone and unattended, for being mischievous, but in a delightful way.

Tutors came and went but her therapist came every week during Linda's childhood and teenage years. Her stay at Chapin Hospital was not without problems. There were so many children to treat, and the hospital was not adequately staffed. One treatment prescribed was hot compresses, which by the time they were applied to Linda's limbs were not hot or even warm, but cold. When a consulting orthopedic doctor examined her at our request, he determined that her legs and arms were stiff and painful. He suggested that we take Linda home where she could have more fitting treatment. We willingly followed his instructions.

But the compresses were far from the end of the treatment. Linda's legs needed reconstructive surgery. Three operations were required so she could be fitted with braces that would enable her to walk a little with the use of crutches. But for the most part, she spent her childhood and the rest of her life confined to a wheelchair. While her body was limited, her mind was not. Maybe it was the inability to move freely, to play as other children played, that was in part responsible for a mind that developed well beyond her years. I can remember being bombarded with questions that I was at times hard-put to answer. She demanded more and more books to read, not the usual childhood fare, but books that imparted information which took her well beyond her wheelchair and into a universe full of mystery. I remember when she first read a copy of Scientific American. She could not put the magazine down. I decided to order a subscription.

As mentioned earlier, Linda had been tutored in our house. It was now time for her to attend school, not a school for children physically impaired, but a school attended by the youngsters in our town. I was apprehensive and perhaps too protective. I worried about how the children would react to someone in a wheelchair. I worried how Linda would react when she found that she could not play the games that other children played.

I soon discovered that there was no need to worry. The first day of school, the children gathered around my daughter and began asking questions. They wanted to know about her ability to move so quickly, how she managed going up and down the aisles. She was more than willing to share the secrets of her success. When they played games, they made Linda a member of the team by appointing her scorekeeper and then later referee. She was more than adequate in performing the tasks assigned. Her score sheet became a badge of honor. She looked forward to the volleyball games as much as the most successful players. Our daughter was popular not because she was handicapped, but because she was a contributing member of her class.

It was during Linda's years in school that George and I realized that our daughter could possibly have a full, rich life. The grade school years passed quickly. Then junior high followed in an accessible new facility. She continued her education in public school. Her choice was classical college, which meant four years of math, physics, English, history, and two languages. She chose Latin and French.

We were a family no different from any other family. We celebrated the holidays. Christmas especially was a time of joy and laughter. We decorated a tree and were careful to pick the right presents for our children. Linda had asked for a microscope and Peter seemed pleased with the model cars we selected.

In high school, Linda excelled first in algebra, then in geometry, and in the fourth year, trigonometry and an elementary introduction to calculus. All her young life she had loved reading, not only scientific magazines, but the classics, which so many of the young had found a bore.

She participated fully in extracurricular activities, and at the insistence of her classmates, she attended school dances. I recognized that my daughter was by nature an observer. She could watch her young friends dancing and did so without envy. In fact, she was intrigued by young bodies in motion. What propelled people into walking the way they did, speaking the way they did, thinking the way they did? She committed to paper her observations. And not unlike many philosophers, she was intrigued by the human condition. Envy was not part of her vocabulary. Her days were filled with 'whys' about everything with the exception of her own physical condition.

She had been committing to paper her observations almost from the time she had learned to write. As the years passed, she developed an understanding not only of herself, but of the people with whom she came in contact. She was more than ready for college. It came as no surprise that she announced that she wanted to be a pre-med student, not because she would one day find a remedy for her own condition, but rather by the desire to alleviate the suffering of those less fortunate.

Linda certainly was no saint, nor did she suffer from a martyr complex, but she was indeed remarkable. If she ever felt sorry for herself, in the early years and in the later years, she never gave voice to lamenting her condition. It was almost as if she realized that her time was limited. She could not waste it on self-pity.

As I mentioned earlier, Linda loved New York. She selected NYU as the medical institution she wished to attend, not only because of location, but because, like Barnard, the medical school had dormitories that were easily accessible to classrooms, labs and libraries. She loved the school and readily bonded with her classmates, admittedly more with the men than women. She found that they were as intense as she was and selected medicine, not because it would insure riches, but because they had an overwhelming desire to come to the aid of their fellow men. With the training acquired and their natural ability, they were prepared to do battle. That was the way Linda thought of her chosen profession- a battle against disease, a battle to save lives, a battle to better the human condition.

She bonded with her microscope, a constant companion in her chosen field—hematology. It seemed that from the beginning of her medical studies, she knew that she would choose that field, and never once doubted that she had made the right decision. Upon completion of internship and residency at New York University Medical Center, she joined a small group of hematologists. She, without hesitation, rejected the recommendations of some of her professors. They strongly urged that she work with paraplegics. She had no interest in doing so. When she told me about the pressure to work in physical medicine, she told me that all her life she had "stood on her own two feet" and she said this with laughter. "You know what I mean, Mom. I considered hematology the cutting edge of medicine. When you think of what can be discovered from blood, the most magnificent diagnostic tool of all medicine, then for me there is no other choice."

Throughout her working life, she lived in the same apartment building on Twenty Third Street, but not in the same apartment. Her small salary forced her to share an apartment, but later, when she had a practice of her own, she could afford living alone. A cleaning woman came in once a week, but that was all the help she had. She had long ago learned to bathe herself, dress herself, no different from any young woman not confined to a wheelchair. When she looked back on her days at NYU, she realized that she was the only student in a wheelchair, but she was never granted special privileges.

Time passed quickly. She was at last seeing patients who were anemic, patients with leukemia that forced her to add oncology as one of her important disciplines. The turning point in her career came when a young flight attendant flying for Canadian Airlines called for an appointment. Upon examination, she noticed purple lesions on his neck. The lesions were different from any she had ever seen. She asked the young man about his itinerary, where he had last flown. The first thought that came to mind was some rare tropical skin disease. The young man had not flown to Africa or South America or India. His general routine was flights to Paris. As the months passed, no medicine seemed to work. Upon each examination, the lesions had increased, not only increased but also multiplied.

"I have a case," she told me on one of her visits home, "and it's extremely challenging. My patient has these purple spots that keep spreading and there's nothing I can do about it. Nothing I've tried works." In little over a year, the young man had died. Within a short period of time, other patients were referred to Linda and they too had lesions. It did not take our daughter long to determine that some strange and heretofore unknown malady was attacking young men. While not always readily discernable, she realized that some of the men were homosexuals. "All right," she said, "so they're gay and I say 'so what'." The light was beginning to dawn.

When her patient died, Linda kept asking herself why. The fact that she had no treatment was a torment. As time passed, there were other patients, patients with lesions she was unable to treat, lesions that multiplied and defied explanation or cure. Then, the word was out that my daughter was treating young men with a disease that was new, that was different, that was deadly. At first, there was not the realization that lesions seemed to be confined to men, and more specifically gay men. The death toll mounted and so many of the victims were writers, musicians, actors. As the cases increased, many doctors, fearful that they might become infected, sent patients to Linda who seemed to have no fear. Before long, she realized that the new disease could possibly be of pandemic proportions restricted not to New York City, not to the United States, but worldwide. Linda and her colleagues determined that the heart of the problem was the relationship between casual sex and the growing number of cases.

7

After questioning her patients and getting them to talk about brief encounters, Linda realized that the bathhouses of New York played no small part in the spread of the disease. She enlisted some of her patients and doctors to prevail upon the mayor of New York at the time, Ed Koch, to close the bathhouses, but to no avail. Many of the young men resented the intrusion and the questioning of their lifestyles. Papers were written and published in the medical journals. The eighties turned into the nineties, and Linda was dismayed that the U.S. government, presidents and congressmen were unwilling to face the fact that a plague was in the land; prejudice, not understanding, ruled the day.

Others have told the story far better than I can. Many of Linda's patients became her friends. She entertained them in her apartment. She refused to have an unlisted phone number and visited the victims day and night, always alone in her wheelchair. She paid no attention to the price she had to pay—always seeking an answer, always trying to impart courage to the young men as they faced death.

Linda bought a house on Cape Cod. It was there that she retreated for a brief respite from AIDs, from the inattention of the whole country. She had her flowers and her two cats, Pumpkin and Cosby, and the friendship of the patients and doctors and her family to sustain her.

Her lungs were never strong, and an asthmatic condition had plagued her for a lifetime. Finally on one of her Cape Cod visits, she was unable to breathe. She was put in an iron lung at the Cape Cod Hospital. I cried; George was beside himself. Seeing Linda once more confined to an iron lung was as painful as the time when she was five years old. Miraculously, she survived and went back to her practice.

I like to think that Linda died just of a coronary, not of a broken heart—a broken heart because she was one of the early discoverers of a deadly disease and was unable to find a cure. Her funeral was held in Harwich, Massachusetts, a small town on Cape Cod. So many of the doctors with whom she had worked so courageously were in attendance.

This is not my story, but Linda's story. I have asked friends she knew to write tales about my daughter. They are childhood friends, college friends, medical school colleagues, and patients. I consider what they wrote to be the most important part of this publication—

Tales of Linda—for which I thank all who have so willingly put into writing their memories of my daughter.

A LOVE LETTER
I LIVE WITH LINDA EVERY DAY

Larry Kramer

I have been in love with Dr. Linda Laubenstein ever since 1981 when she became my doctor. I have been living with Linda since 1983 when I started writing my play, The Normal Heart, in which she is one of the leading characters. I am still living with her now that the movie of my play is about to begin shooting. I have been able, because it is a movie, to greatly expand her part, which will be played by Julia Roberts. Ellen Barkin, who played Emma in the Broadway production, received a Tony for her portrayal of Linda. Over all these years since the play first opened in 1984, it has been done all over America and all over the world. Hundreds of actresses by now have played her. Linda would never come and see the play when it was first done at the Public Theater here in New York, even though our producer, Joseph Papp, offered to send a limousine. I of course gave her a copy of the play before we ever did anything, but she told me she wouldn't read it. I'm uncertain why she felt this way. Someone suggested it might be because there were also other doctors at New York University Medical Center who were also taking care of patients who had what would become known as AIDS. And that by singling her out, she felt I might be exploiting her because she was in a wheelchair, and hence more dramatic. I confess to being guilty of this. I wanted to make a parallel with her courage in overcoming such a physical liability as a yardstick for the guys getting sick to see what courage can really be. The play is still being produced everywhere and with the movie, all of which is accompanied with the information that the part of Dr. Emma Brookner is based on Dr. Linda Laubenstein, will, I hope, enshrine her legacy forever. I miss her very much. Her courage gave me courage, a great gift.

My Memories of Linda

Barbara Waterman

The Memorial Service at the First Congregational Church in Harwich, Massachusetts was certainly a celebration of the life of Linda J. Laubenstein. Her memory and good work will always be an integral part of the world. However, I didn't know her as Dr. Laubenstein; I knew her as a friend of over 40 years and by the name of Dee-Dah. I remember the holidays, funerals, sicknesses, and weddings we shared with Linda and her family. A holiday gathering of both families included T-Dot, Nana Martin, Grampa, Moo-Moo, and Lola. The cat who was appropriately named by Linda as Lola got whatever Lola wanted including the entire Christmas turkey. At these gatherings everybody talked at the same time and, of course, always knew more than anybody else. As Linda would say, "A little free advice goes a long way".

I knew Linda before she was afflicted by the terrible virus polio. She was a beautiful little girl who could have adorned the cover of any children's fashion magazine. She was mature then and enjoyed adult company. Her mother called her "Miss Glue". When she got polio, my family was totally absorbed in Linda's well being. If she had a good day, and they were few and far between, we were relieved. If she had a bad day in the iron lung, a very sober, hopeful attitude prevailed. Her parents were at the hospital for long hours for many, many days. Her brother, Peter, was with us a lot.

Linda came home finally. Her father became her back and legs. Her mother was a strong motivational force that would have been impossible for Linda not to pay attention to. Linda would not have made it in any other house.

There were trips to the brace man, Mr. Buschenfeld, and many painful hours with Patsy, the therapist. Patsy and Priscilla would actually make this torture seem worthwhile to Linda. They would tell her all the advantages of this grueling experience and also what would happen if she didn't undergo it.

Linda and I shared a similar plight. We each had pesky little brothers continually doing annoying and embarrassing things to the superior, older sisters. For example, on winter days when the ice melted in a new foundation, Pete and Chris stripped down and went for a swim. Everything was great in this Roman Bath until Mother Laubenstein inadvertently looked out her front window. Jimmy Curren, her neighbor then and mine now, said she bolted from the front door as if she was shot from a cannon. Cold bottoms were very quickly warmed. There ended the Olympian swim but not the humiliation from such a public spectacle. Pete later became Linda's best friend and confidant.

Linda had many subsequent operations. Bones from the legs were put into her back. She would come home and live in a body cast in a hospital bed in the dining room. Only a knitting needle could reach some remote and frequent itches caused by being surrounded in a wall of plaster. Many signatures, drawings, and pungent remarks adorned this rather large cocoon. We played many games with Linda. My brother, George, and Linda were notorious for having 'words' about their many creative interpretations of rules. Both wanted to win all the time. Her mom brought Linda every book from the public library and Linda devoured them much like larvae consume leaves on a tree. It was in this setting that Linda went to school, or rather, it came to her. An intercom was installed on the wall. Mrs. Walkden would say, "Children, open your book to such and such a page, and do such and such." Linda would express her feelings about the lesson and not get into any trouble. There were times she would say that she had enough of that boring lesson and I, the future teacher of 27 years, would shut off the intercom at Linda's bequest. She could actually turn her adversity into something we coveted. Imagine being able to escape lessons and the teacher so easily. She was frequently also known to open a pleasure book or even take a little catnap. From being such an avid reader and frequent eavesdropper on adult conversation, she was precocious enough to not have any gaps in her learning. I have often wondered how many of my little darlings would have shut off my lessons if given the opportunity.

There were no airs about Linda. I never saw her in designer clothes or Italian shoes which she certainly could have afforded. Instead, I saw Dee-Dah in sweat pants, t-shirts after she had burned her bra, and bare feet no matter what the weather. She didn't drive a fancy Mercedes with a car phone. Instead, she donned a beeper and commandeered an electric wheelchair much as though it was an amphibious Jeep. She would go through puddles in the gutter and up and down snow covered sidewalks. I am sure a Mack truck driver would pay attention to this crazy driver.

I didn't know her as a doctor, but as I previously stated, I knew her as Dee-Dah. I once asked her what I should do about my poor sore fingers. She quickly retorted, "Call a doctor." I'm sure she knew I wasn't going to be "carried off" by what she probably considered as serious as a hangnail, and being a Story [family member], I was probably looking for free medical advice.

It was as though she left the doctor part in New York. It was a difficult profession emotionally as well as physically for her. She once confided it was difficult to treat someone for a long time and then lose him through no fault of her own. She had just lost a young boy. What goes around comes around. Just like her patients, she was given great care and devotion, and tragically and helplessly succumbed.

However, Linda did not die in vain. With people like Linda, we will some day have a world free of AIDS, Patsies, Mr. Buschenfields, iron lungs, ostentation, hypocrisy, and unemployment. Sometimes it is hard to see these overall implications. The hard reality is that we have lost a beloved member of our extended family.

Dee Dah up Close

Barbara Waterman

The Iron Lung is a perfect metaphor for Linda Jane Laubenstein. In spite of multiple handicaps she kept moving towards her ambitious goals. Her legs dangled freely when someone picked her up. She used her right arm by guiding it with her left arm. Her body cast served as an outward manifestation of an inward strength. I used to secretly smuggle a knitting needle to scratch the inside of her cast. She would give out a great sigh of relief. Where there is a will, there is a way. In this case the will power was overwhelming.

The setting for this was the family dining room. Here she was hooked up to her classroom at Nayatt School by an intercom. Many times she would say, "Let's shut it off." Her teacher, Mrs. Walkden, the epitome of a dedicated teacher would bring Linda hot lunches. This was well and fine until she came into the dining room and found the intercom off and Linda and her cat, Lola, having a catnap.

One time I brought Linda a peach shortcake. We laughed hysterically when it dawned on us the owner of the peach trees must have been too frugal to spray. A worm wiggled up through the whipped cream and waved his body at Linda. I will especially never forget the tuft of whipped cream on this creature's head and the look of horror on Linda's face. This was only a temporary reaction. She removed the creature and ate the shortcake. Like in all of life, nothing deterred her.

Extraordinary

Karen Wells Washley

Surprisingly, I am finding it more difficult than I ever thought to articulate my memories of my childhood neighbor and pal Linda Laubenstein. It may be that I was so young at the time we were living across the street from one another, it could have been that she was part of my daily life that I took for granted or it could be that I had a terrible memory.

I do know that at that time when I was 7 through 13 years old, Linda always seemed so much older, wiser and more mature than I did, although she was only a year older than I. She lived in a well-regulated world of medical procedures and adults. I felt very privileged and important to have been invited to visit her in the hospital or to have been the one chosen to help her with visiting the school rest room. There was a bit of an idea in my mind that she was extra special, and that I was lucky to be the close-by girl, who knew her well.

My first overnight at a girlfriend's house was at Linda's home. She had nifty twin beds that were up against the wall at right angles, making lights-out conversation a little more difficult. But an overnight just doesn't work without being able to whisper your secrets through the dark. Oh, how I wish I could recollect what made us laugh enough to have feared her parents coming in and hushing us. To reciprocate bedroom visits, one day Linda came to my home, and my mother and I brought her up to my second floor room. I hate to think how battered she must have been by our pulling her up the stairs one at a time, with her braces most likely clunking against the treads. The treasures within my bedroom awaited, and I was very determined to have my friend see my book, toy, doll and perfume collections.

Long before Barbie dolls were popular, Linda and I played with Ginny dolls. They were sweet shapeless dolls that encouraged little girls to use their imaginations to create scenes and conversations for their little friends. We dressed them in their colorful outfits, some made by mothers, babysitters or ourselves, and filled hours with the chatter girls have—lost in the endless fun of playing with their favorite dolls. Those dolls must have drunk hundreds of little cups of tea and eaten cookies well beyond their snack allotment. In thinking back upon those times I realized what a carefree and innocent period it was in our lives and how wonderful it was to have had the vehicle of dolls to express ourselves and create lives beyond our homes.

Linda was special; I just did not know at the time that she was extraordinary.

BRISTOL FOURTH OF JULY PARADE

Tom Doyle

Dear Terry,

In talking to Priscilla Laubenstein last evening, I learned you were the family's minister, and also that you and I attended Brown very close to the same time. You graduated in 1962, a year before I. Priscilla reflected how life has surprising turns. Our somewhat coincidental acquaintance is a pleasant turn. And the occasion for my learning of you in the first place is that I understand you will be doing the memorial service for Linda this Saturday. Her sudden departure from us is a surprising turn, indeed.

The Laubensteins included me in their family during my freshman summer. I lived in their home in Barrington. George would drive to work for Providence Gas Co., and drop me off where I could walk to the campus for my summer job in the botany lab. I worked for Dr. Mel Fuller in Rogers Hall.

Peter and Linda were the kids at home. I think I grew up more than they did, being exposed to the lives of the Laubenstein family.

Linda was a remarkable human being, and remains a remarkable influence in my life. I do not know how well you knew her. By knowing her parents, though, you knew her to a degree. In them is a righteous insistence. Priscilla would never allow Linda to back off of that position. Yes, she was gifted. In a lesser person, coming from lesser parents, her gifts could have turned inward to self-pity. Linda, I say to myself, died because she was tired out for having lived so intensely—giving herself. George said she left 32 patients in the hospital. From what I remember of his prior descriptions of her work, that was a fairly typical caseload. It was only a portion of her workday.

But you will hear many examples of this kind of living about Linda. You and others will marvel at her accomplishments, as I. There is an incident, though, I will relate to say something of the very personal.

Priscilla's direction to me on that Fourth of July, 1960, was to take Linda to the parade at Bristol. So I loaded up the wheelchair and Linda in the little Morris Minor the family had. It was equipped with a rack on the back for the wheelchair. I had, by then, learned how to position the wheelchair and to do what Linda needed while she would scoot herself to and from the car seat to the wheel chair. She, by then, had become like a kid sister to me, so I would do what family does— get the job done and get on with life. The wheelchair, the braces, and all of the procedure became a kind of parenthesis, while the focus of the day was the parade.

Have you ever been to a New England town for such a parade? I cannot remember many details. There is a general impression of color and music and continually changing attractions passing before us, with the folks along the street side having as good a time as those in the parade. Truly, nothing singularly remarkable happened that day but for the indelible impression, from then on, of how Linda was. She was a deeply happy person. The word is too misunderstood—happy. But when I think of the word, Linda defines it for me. We both worked through all of the parenthesis business. The focus of why we were there was the joy of the special day. She'd fuss and pout as any growing girl would do, yet that was just another parenthesis she had to get through for her to get back to the focus of her life. I now recall a verse which helps us with the way to focus: "Looking unto Jesus the author and finisher of our faith; who for the job that was set before him endured the cross, despising the shame, and is set down at the right hand of the throne of God." She looked at joy set before her.

Linda could see what others did not see. Her parents can also see in this way. Thus their influence. I thank God for that influence on me, as well.

So I have Linda hidden in my heart as a smiling young girl. Such was my blessing to have enjoyed her at that time in her life. As I said to Peter, "I had the best years with her." Others who knew her as a physician will treasure her as a dear physician, and that is as it should be. For me, I am happy I have her as, with the little smile and twinkle in her eye, she would have me, smiling back at her at this very moment. And, of course, I weep as I do so, for she is gone from us for a while.

I know your heart and soul will bless the Saturday coming. You've got an awesome job. How can you improve on the sunshine? I guess by being happy for it's shining so golden and warm. Thus, Linda Laubenstein, sunshine.

Warm regards and more,

Tom Doyle.

FLEEING THE IRON CURTAIN

Vera Albanesi

Dr. Linda Laubenstein's practice at NYU was really busy when in
1981 she hired a 32-year-old stranger from what was then 'behind'
the Iron Curtain to help out in the office. No qualms about the fact the
stranger spoke broken English, that she was not familiar with the
medical practice, insurance and other routines in the United States so
it would have been a no-brainer to go for someone else. But I was
hired and although I left after two years for personal reasons, we
became friends and saw each other often until she passed away in her
beloved cottage in Cape Cod.

In a way Linda seems to have been born somehow fated for the
role her professional life shoed her into. Her steely character elevated
her to parity with any other human being, but her sincere modesty
rendered Linda accessible to everyone. 'Helped' by a debilitating
disease which gave her a genuine compassion towards the very sick,
and a last name she used to joke "opens doors because people think
I'm Jewish." Linda fit into the role of a pioneer caregiver/researcher
in what became the AIDS epidemic. A difficult role running a
practice where patients were usually lost as Kaposi's sarcoma ate
away at their bodies.

In spite of immersing herself in fighting for her patients, Linda
always had the time for culture. New York's theatres, ballet, museums
and opera provided her therapy and respite from intensive research
and other commitments she undertook at Multitasking Systems, Inc.
(a nonprofit company [she founded] to provide jobs to patients with
AIDS).

I remember one such occasion when we had arranged to meet in
front of the Lincoln Center to see Turandot. The opera started at 8:00
p.m. and we had arranged to meet at 7:30 in front of the Theatre. Cell
phones were barely invented by then and not in much use. No Linda
at 7:30, no Linda at 8:00 and no Linda at 9:00. I called everywhere.
The doorman confirmed Linda had left on time for the theatre. No one

knew where she was. My mind imagined the worst. I have no idea why I decided to wait there for the night, or why Linda decided it was still necessary to get to the theatre even well after 9:00, but there in the distance appeared a little bundle zigzagging around the pedestrians. When she got to me she had no time for niceties and simply said, "Let's go in. It's a long opera." We wheeled in just in time for the intermission and I got the story of Linda's adventure over a glass of champagne. With wheelchair taxis not available, Linda had taken an MTA bus. The bus broke down and the wheelchair mechanism had blocked the doors from opening. The MTA also had no cell phones! And it took forever to get Linda out and to get another wheelchair bus to continue her trip. The champagne really hit the spot and we enjoyed the second half of the evening.

Linda somehow found time. Though home chores and the simple everyday routines took on a different dimension for her, she even took on extra 'selective' chores. When she was told my boyfriend and I were getting married, and knowing all our families were in Europe, with mine still not being able to travel from Eastern Europe, she offered to host our wedding lunch/reception and sent my husband-to-be a "get this act on the road quickly" card, noting there were only three weeks to go. She prepared the menu, invited our friends and basically took care of everything. Linda tended to shun praises but everyone had a ball and when our friends broke out in a genuinely felt thank you chorus of "For she's a jolly good fellow" she was the happiest I had seen in a long time.

At a young 45 years of age, Linda died an accomplished human being who never bragged about climbing the mountains she climbed, who encouraged others to action, and who always had an ear and a solution for everyone else's troubles. At times people found her abrasive, but I prefer my husband's take on that side of Linda. He said she was not abrasive at all. She just had some sort of allergy to idiots. I think it might have been regarding resistance to closing New York's public baths when a reporter asked her if she ever took no for an answer, Linda simply said, "Not if it's not the right answer."

I feel blessed to have had her in my life.

WRATH OF MOTHER

Peter Laubenstein

From an early age, I realized that there was a member of our household who required an inordinate amount of care. When I think back, I am amazed that I had felt no resentment of the attention given my sister Linda. The reason was simple. I loved my sister and hoped that one day she would get out of her wheelchair and play with me.

Consciously or unconsciously, I looked to my sister for companionship because despite caretakers and parents I was essentially alone. I never thought about this condition when I was young and even as an adult. For two people so close, Linda and I were different. Academically, my sister with little effort excelled. I did not. She was by nature a giver, and although I never considered myself a taker, I certainly did not have the welfare of my fellow man of interest or concern. I was not a callous brute but basically no different from most of my fellow men.

Now when I think back, which I seldom do, I am reminded of two incidents that involved Linda and me and my parents. The two episodes were my automobile stories. I always loved automobiles. I can think of no better way of getting from one place to the next on my own and without assistance from a third party.

The first incident involved a young man—Tom Doyle who was in need of inexpensive housing while he attended school. He had sought the help of the Congregational Church and my father and mother decided to give him lodging in our basement, which unlike so many basements, was warm in the winter and far different from the rooms our family occupied. Tom was expected to help my father with the lawn and vegetable garden and perform other chores that were needed. For all these tasks, he was provided meals which he took with the rest of the family and perhaps most important for him the use of a car on the condition he reported his whereabouts and was on time for meals.

I liked Tom. He was the older brother I never had but always wanted. He played games with me. He tried to teach me about automobiles and many other things that came into his head. Perhaps, most important of all, he was willing to spend time with me and never thought it was a chore to do so. At least, that's what I thought at the time.

One evening, my mother had cooked a roast beef dinner, with all the trimmings and she had baked a chocolate cake for dessert. When it was time to sit down for the meal, Tom was absent. And he had failed to call. My mother, always the disciplinarian, became more and more agitated, and we ate our dinner and by the end of the meal, I thought she would explode. Poor Tom, I thought, he's in for big trouble. You don't tangle with Mother.

An hour after we finished eating, Tom arrived. "I lost all track of time," he said. "I'm deeply sorry. I hope you didn't wait dinner for me."

By this time, my mother was livid. "You are an inconsiderate young man," she said. Her voice was like cracked ice. "I'd like to make amends," Tom said. "Why don't I wash the dishes and clean the kitchen." Mother didn't bother answering. Father then decided to get into the act. "That would be very nice, Tom," Father said.

We all went to sit in the living room. Mother said nothing. Linda looked at me and I looked at Linda. We both felt bad that Tom had met with such disfavor. Father pulled out his pipe but refrained from smoking. We could hear the banging of pots and pans. And then silence.

We waited for Tom to finish in the kitchen, and an inordinate length of time seemed to pass. At last Tom joined us in the living room. We took one look at him and determined that something was amiss. Tom was covered with white bubbles that were streaming down his face and covered his trousers.

"I don't know what went wrong," he said. I thought for a minute he was going to cry. "I don't know what went wrong," he said again.

Father moved toward the kitchen. Linda wheeled into the kitchen and I followed Linda. Only Mother held back. The kitchen floor was covered with suds and suds were streaming out of the dishwasher. Father took off his shoes, I took off my shoes and the two of us waded into the mess. Linda's feet did not touch the floor. On top of the sink,

Father spotted a container of Ivory soap liquid, not dishwasher fluid but Ivory soap. He burst out laughing and Linda began laughing and only Tom did not participate. "I'm so sorry," he said. "I'm so sorry. Give me time to clean up this mess."

Finally Mother entered the kitchen. She saw Father holding the Ivory soap container and she too began to laugh. Tom, holding a mop and pail in his hands, promised that he would never again forget to call. And much to Linda's relief and my relief and Father's relief, Mother forgave all. Tom was allowed to stay and continued to drive the car.

To the Rescue

Peter Laubenstein

I was already an adult when my next automobile story took place. Throughout my teenage years, I lived without purpose and, frankly, without caring about succeeding. One achiever in the family was enough. I could not take credit for Linda making it through med school and becoming the doctor she always wanted to be. But her success was no incentive to me. It took a long time for me to decide what I wanted to do, a long time, despite the prodding from my parents, which was always a bore rather than an incentive. They were not successful in trying to get into my head. Secretly I thought their trying to do so was a joke. I guess that from early on I was a drifter, drifting from school to school, from subject to subject. I attended college in the South, far away from the cold and rigidity of New England. I had my own car, and the wheels enabled me to break away from school and from studying whenever I became too depressed. I loved my little automobile. It represented freedom.

Late one afternoon I decided to drive as far as I could. I didn't have a destination in mind. Maybe that was descriptive of my whole way of life.

I found myself driving at a reasonable speed. I was in territory that was unfamiliar, but that was more interesting than fearful. I can't remember how many hours I was on the road. I felt my eyes closing momentarily every now and then. But it never occurred to me that I was dozing off, that I was, in fact, in danger of falling asleep at the wheel. And then the unthinkable happened. Almost without warning, I found myself in a deep pile of mud. The front to the car was smashed and it was a miracle that I wasn't killed.

Sheer panic set in. I wasn't hurt. Only my self-esteem had gone down a notch or two. It occurred to me that it would have been a fitting ending if I had been killed. At least I would be free of having to make decisions about what I should do with my life. I had long ago given up pleasing my parents. My mother was anxious for me to write my tale. I know she'll be appalled when she reads this. But so be it.

I managed to get out of the car. Cell phones were not in use. I stood knee deep in the mud and was unable to think about what my next move should be. Somehow or other, I reached the road and prayed that some car would come along. After what seemed like hours, a sleek sedan was moving down the road. I reached for a handkerchief in my pocket and began waving it in my hands. I stood smack in the middle of the road. I knew the driver would have to stop because the road was too narrow for him to skirt around me. Fortunately, he did stop. Without saying a word, I pointed to my totaled car, which had sunken further into the mud.

We didn't really speak to each other. I asked my rescuer to drop me off in the next town so that I could telephone for help. Fortunately, I had money in my pocket. When I got out of the car, I offered him a few dollars. He shook his head and went on his way. A local drugstore was open. I spotted a telephone down the aisle and asked permission to use it.

I didn't call my parents. My first and only thought was to call Linda.

When she answered, I blurted out, "Linda, I totaled my car. No I'm all right. Could you wire me money so I can buy another set of wheels?"

There was no hesitation at her end.

"Of course, Peter. Are you sure you're all right?"

We worked out the details. Within a few hours the money arrived. I never stopped to think why I had called Linda and not my parents. Maybe it was because I wasn't in the mood for a lecture. Maybe because I feared they would not send the money. Maybe it was because of an even greater fear—that they would fly down and drag me home. All I knew then, and what I know now is that in my moment of distress and feeling completely alone in the world, I turned to the one I loved more than any other human being I loved and trusted—my sister Linda.

STRENGTH OF CHARACTER

Dr. Jeffrey Martin

"I am part of all I have seen."—Lord Alfred Tennyson

Many accomplished individuals can point to one or two people who have had a major impact on their life. For me that special mentor was my cousin, Linda Laubenstein. Linda was an amazing woman whose strength of character served as an inspiration for me in my medical career. Over the years I have reflected on the values that were instilled in me by watching her deal with daily challenges—both professionally and as an individual.

I never viewed Linda as having a handicap nor would she ever allow herself to be viewed that way. She dealt with her physical limitations with the mantra of "adapt and overcome." The few times I visited Linda in NYC, I had a hard time keeping up with her—she knew the city and it seemed everyone in her neighborhood knew her well. She indeed was a Renaissance woman and her love of art, theater, literature and music was obvious to all that knew her. She brought this love of life to all those for whom she cared, including and especially her patients.

I was at a personal crossroad during the mid-eighties and, in retrospect, I looked to Linda as my signpost. I wasn't fully aware of Linda's research and work with HIV patients until I began to speak with her about my experiences as an anesthetist at Emory University. I had just completed my master's at Emory University School of Medicine and had begun work with the Department of Anesthesiology, Division of Cardiothoracic Anesthesia. We were starting to see patients coming to the O.R. for lung biopsies on suspicious pulmonary lesions. Many of these patients had experienced unexplained dramatic weight loss, fevers, fatigue and coughs that were unresponsive to current medical therapies. I was not fully aware of what it meant to be diagnosed with HIV/AIDS as this was just coming to the forefront of medicine. Little did I realize, that in Linda,

I had the opportunity of a lifetime to learn from one of the pioneers in AIDS research and it wasn't until after I was in medical school did I realize just how important her research work in the HIV/AIDS community was. Some of her research papers were required reading while I was in medical school.

Linda did much for my understanding of the emerging epidemic and allowed me a special insight to the physical and psychological needs for this special group of patients. Along the way Linda's compassion and academic curiosity instilled a greater sense of wonder for me in medicine.

Linda touched many lives and in ways that I can never fully appreciate, except in my own circumstance. I will always be grateful for Linda's encouragement for me to pursue my dreams and for her strength in facing life's challenges while pursuing her dreams.

Opportunity Knocks

Donna Destefano Griffin

On January 1, 1979, I boarded the train in Providence, Rhode Island, lugging one suitcase and a guitar and feeling both apprehensive and exhilarated by the possibilities ahead. At age 28, I was recovering from a failed romance and grateful for the opportunity for a fresh start—a new job, new digs, new life in—ta da—New York! That is how Linda and I became friends.

We grew up in the same town and when Linda was at Barnard, my family coincidentally moved right across the street from hers. However, the four-year age difference had kept us in separate schools and our paths did not cross until Linda's first year as an attending physician. Actually, it was our respective mothers who instigated the journey.

Linda was sharing an office with two other physicians and they were all in desperate need of an office manager. Linda probably complained to her mother. I complained to my mother that I needed a job and a change of scenery. My mother met her mother in the grocery store and a few weeks later I was awestruck in Grand Central Station.

Linda lived on the 22nd floor of a doorman building on East 25th Street, one block west of "bed pan alley", a row of hospitals along twenty blocks of First Avenue. It was a one-bedroom apartment with wrap around terrace where Jake, the twenty pound cat, would exit his special door to visit the litter box. Linda invited me to stay with her until I'd saved up enough money to get my own place. I slept on a cot in her living room for a year. She would accept no rent. In return, my job was to feed Jake, a ritual that began at 6:00 every morning with Jake pouncing on my chest and resting his wet nose between my eyes.

Jake was a very cool cat and unique as his mistress. He would wait by the door when he heard the key in the lock and give us each a kiss when we returned home for the day. Once when Linda took him to her house in Chatham for the weekend, the baggage handlers forgot to take him off the plane on the return trip to New York and he flew on to San Francisco. He was delivered to our building by limousine, calm and self-assured as ever.

It was great fun living with Linda. She loved to cook and was very good at it. Her terrace garden was magnificent, blooming in summer with the most robust petunias I'd ever seen. Linda shared her love of reading, ballet, live theater and movies and taught me how to get around the city—which is rather ironic since I was the able bodied person.

In the 1980's, several theaters offered serious discounts for people using wheelchairs. One person escorting them also received a discounted ticket. We saw many great shows together. I remember the night we went to see Cats. It was raining when we exited the theater, and people were snatching cabs from me each time I turned to position Linda's chair so I could lift her into the cab and then toss the chair in the trunk. I finally had to walk two blocks from the theater to secure a cab, bribing the cabby to stop and wait until we picked up Linda and not, in the interim, to take off with another fare. Although getting progressively drenched, Linda remained her usual patient self, praising my resourcefulness and finding humor in the situation.

When her friend from medical school who lived on the 18th floor in our building got a job in California, Linda helped me move into his apartment. We shopped together for furniture and Linda shared her gardening secrets for beautifying my terrace. When another friend was leaving a job she thought I would like, Linda got me an interview. When I got pneumonia, she nursed me back to health. She encouraged me to further my education and often discussed her philosophy of medicine and patient care as if talking with a colleague of equal intellectual stature. A person interacting with Linda would feel respect, validation and empathy.

Linda had amazing personal fortitude. The most basic activities of daily living presented challenges that would confound many in her situation, but she approached life with gusto and determination that was awe-inspiring. Her accomplishments as a scientist and physician are remarkable; as a severe asthmatic and paraplegic, they are epic. But to me, Linda was a kind, generous, funny, supportive and loving soul who always gave me a helping hand when I needed it most.

I wish that I could say that I truly appreciated Linda's authenticity when we were roommates and neighbors, but that would be untrue. Joni Mitchell's words from Big Yellow Taxi come to mind:

"Don't it always seem to go

That we don't know what we've got 'til it's gone..."

Perhaps if the spirit that is Linda Laubenstein had been blessed with a healthier body her impact upon the world would not have been as powerful. By her learning to transcend her physical disabilities, Linda has taught us all not to underestimate her potential, to strive for excellence, to persevere and to care for others. Linda's time with us was a precious gift to the world.

Weekend in Barrington

Pamela Gallagher

Linda couldn't walk but she sure got around. She cruised the Barnard campus in her battery-powered wheelchair and used her standard one for traveling around the city. She would grab a pal or two and we would go to the museums, Broadway, shopping, out to restaurants or the New York City Ballet. Under her patient teaching, we were all adept at hailing a cab, getting her into it and stowing her wheelchair in the trunk.

Off campus, we would pile into a car and take off. Trips to Barrington, RI to visit Linda and her parents usually revolved around a summer activity. The summer after we graduated college, I got married and Linda prepared for medical school. Paul, my new husband, was in the Army and stationed at Ft. Devens, the only army base in New England. That summer, we took off every weekend going to Vermont to visit my family, Armonk, NY to visit his or to Cape Cod. On the weekend of the Newport Folk Festival, July 19th, we stayed with Linda and her family in Barrington.

What a weekend that turned out to be! We drove up Friday, July 18th, relaxed over dinner and made plans for a picnic in Newport before the festival the next day. Waking up the next morning we were greeted at breakfast with the news of Teddy Kennedy and the horrible events of Chappaquiddick. We were stunned. Priscilla, Linda's mother, grew up in and around Boston and had plenty to say about how she and her friends were warned by their mothers to stay away from those Kennedy boys. The TV showed non-stop videos and pictures of all things Kennedy—a pre-curser to the 24-hour news cycle we have all come to know.

However, we had a concert to attend. We packed the picnic, loaded up the car, and took off for Newport. We dined in a park overlooking the water. The three of us chatted about who was performing, where to park, and the events of the past 24 hours. By the time we got to the festival grounds and parked, we looked for space to watch the concert. Naturally, because we showed up later than most, we wound up far, far away from the stage. What a night. Arlo Guthrie headlined the show. So many performers under a beautiful summer night. While we couldn't see too much (the stage was so far away), we sure could hear the music.

Sunday, the papers were full of all the Chappaquiddick news, rumors and speculations. More talk around the breakfast table, more disbelief about how something could go so wrong, sadness for the woman who lost her life.

Before Paul and I headed back to Ft. Devens, Linda and her folks treated us to an old-fashioned clambake. As we all pitched in to get it ready, news of Neil Armstrong and Buzz Aldrin landing on the moon broke into the news stream. We were glued to the images of the landing and the preparation for their walk the next day. Before we left, we all knew we had shared a very special segment of time when many disparate forces came together over a summer weekend in New England.

Over the years, we met up with Linda mostly in New York City. As our family grew, we introduced them to Aunt Linda. I have a picture in my mind of Linda in her motorized wheelchair holding our youngest in her arms while our son was playing with the controls and making her go in circles. Our older daughter just hung on to the chair trying to get a word in edgewise while her brother talked non-stop.

Our final memory of Linda again is in New York. We met her at her apartment and took her out to dinner at Union Square Café. It had recently opened and was the hot restaurant in the city. Linda booked the reservations well in advance. She recommended the blackened tuna rare; it was divine. As we were leaving we made plans to meet on the Cape at her house in Chatham. We offered to walk her back to her apartment that was in the neighborhood. She said that wasn't necessary. She was on her home turf. We said good night and watched her cruise away.

ON THE NORMAL HEART

Dr. Richard Ostreicher

To my knowledge, Linda never saw Larry Kramer's The Normal Heart, although she knew that she was the inspiration for a major sympathetic, even heroic, character. Many of her friends and acquaintances have speculated, some in print, why this was so. I have heard that she did not wish to view herself wheelchair-bound, much as Franklin D. Roosevelt avoided having photographs taken that included his wheelchair. I don't think, however, that this was really the case. Linda was an immensely private and modest person who, I believe, was somewhat embarrassed by the notoriety of being seen as a modern day Joan of Arc. She was content to stay in the background, caring for her patients when others would not, working outside of the medical setting to find meaningful employment for her patients when they lost their jobs due to fear and prejudice, and working behind the scenes to raise money for patient home care and AIDS research.

As much as she admired Larry Kramer's work and came to love him as a friend, she told me that he could be a real "pain in the butt". Others, Larry Kramer included, would not be quite so polite. Linda felt that Larry was pressuring her to assume a public role that she felt was "unprofessional" given her New England upbringing and reserve. She found it hard to be in the spotlight, even if the character was named "Emma". She was Linda nevertheless in courage, spirit, and intelligence.

Still, she read and was impressed with the script and loved that Larry had the guts to show what she and her colleagues knew (but what the media and politicians ignored): AIDS was destroying our New York gay community and would certainly find its way to the population at large.

We had a great deal of fun regarding the casting of the play when it was announced to be part of the Public Theatre's season. We'd come up with all sorts of wild casting possibilities for the character of Emma, ranging from Farrah Fawcett to Katherine Hepburn! For her part, Linda was hoping for Emma to be played by someone with "class" who could, at least, act, assuming that Miss Hepburn would be otherwise engaged. We had seen The Year of Living Dangerously around the same time and had both been intrigued with Linda Hunt. She won the Academy Award for her performance and actually bore a strong resemblance to Linda. Linda mentioned at one point that Linda Hunt would probably be ideal for the part, but given the need for a "star", the part would probably go to someone with "tits and glitter".

Imagine her reaction, when Larry Kramer informed her that Barbra Streisand was interested in the film rights and might even take on the part of Emma herself! We had a good laugh about it and she said, "She'd better clip her damn nails if she's going to do a rectal!"

A FRIEND ON BROADWAY: THE NORMAL HEART

Hallie Ephron

Tomorrow night is the Broadway opening for Larry Kramer's searing drama The Normal Heart. It's about the early days of the AIDS epidemic, and I only wish that my friend Dr. Linda Laubenstein … could be there to see it.

One of the play's main characters, Dr. Emma Brookner, is a smart, caring, take-no-prisoners physician who has been confined to a wheelchair since she contracted childhood polio. Emma Brookner is based on Linda. Linda was also my roommate at Barnard College and a dear friend.

The Normal Heart ran for years off-Broadway in the '80s and since in various productions. Dr. Emma Brookner has been played by, among others, actresses Julie Harris, Barbara Bel Geddes, Joanna Gleason, and Judith Lightfoot. Barbara Streisand optioned the play for years, planning to play the role herself in a film version.

Now, on Broadway at last, Ellen Barkin steps into the role; Joe Mantello plays Ned Weeks, the character based on Larry Kramer; Joel Grey directs.

I met Linda the day I arrived from California as a freshman at Barnard College in 1965. She was attractive and slim with straight brown hair cut in bangs, and big features- large, expressive brown eyes and a toothy smile that took over her face. From years of physical therapy, her shoulders were muscular; from a summer spent on Cape Cod her skin was the color of coffee with cream in it. Despite multiple operations, her back was twisted. Her legs, encased in steel braces, were delicate and child-like. Among other things, we shared a subscription to the New York City Ballet.

I never intended to become friends with Linda. I have no patience with people who can't keep up. It turned out, neither did Linda.

She went on to complete her MD at NYU in 1973, became a hematologist, and in 1979 she was at the heart of the early discovery of AIDS. She was the first among her profession to hear the name

Gaetan Dugas, the flight attendant who would become known as "Patient Zero", the friend and common denominator to both of the first gay men patients whom she saw with unusual cancerous lesions. She organized the first medical conference on AIDS, and developed a groundbreaking chemotherapy regimen, a so-called AIDS cocktail, that prolonged lives.

In the 1980s, Linda got to know Larry Kramer, the outspoken writer and activist who organized the Gay Men's Health Cooperative and the more radical ACT UP. She treated his partner and many of his friends, making house calls via New York City transit buses. When they died, as they all did, she went to their funerals.

Over the decade of their friendship, Kramer told me that he became Linda's voice, and she became his conscience. She didn't mind that he wrote a play about her, but he once told me she was furious that he'd put her character in a wheelchair. She refused to attend even a single performance.

Linda died suddenly in 1992. I wish she'd seen The Normal Heart because her friend Larry really did justice to her and all of her anger, despair, and passion. I wish I could be there Wednesday with Linda's mother Priscilla and her brother Peter, and to congratulate Larry Kramer, still alive against all odds, when the play opens at the John Golden Theatre on West 45th Street.

Wow, Hallie, that's an amazing story! Those were terrible times and this sounds like a must-see. And what a powerful group of women have played that part—I would love to see Ellen Barkin in this role.

Thanks for the detour!
R.I.

What a terrific story, Hallie. Depart more often, there is nothing more inspiring than a story about a real, life hero - heroine.
J.B.

Wow, thank you Hallie, talk about a powerful woman.
H.P.R.

I have a feeling she knows all about it.
P.S.

She really was pretty amazing. Tough, funny. At the hospital she was known somewhat uncharitably as "hell on wheels" because she demanded what she needed for her patients.
Hallie Ephron

Many thanks, Hallie, for diverting from the usual today. This has special significance for me, as a dear friend was the first AIDS victim to die here in Cincinnati. None of us had even heard of the disease at that time, and he and his partner had never actually said they were gay (but we who loved them knew). We still miss him terribly, too.

Thank goodness for courageous doctors like Linda, for her tireless dedication to curing this awful affliction.
K.

Wow, Hallie, I'd love to see this, especially with Ellen Barkin. Thanks for sharing Linda's story.
D.

Hallie, a good remembrance (sic) and forward look. I remember those early days and they were frightening ... Linda did a ton of good. I didn't know your connection but that is huge. Barkin's interview in last week's NYT shows she brings the right stuff to the role. The play is a reason to get to NY. Thanks for this.
A.D.

This is not a diversion, Hallie. Our blog is about all the elements of our lives, our histories, things that move us, things that matter to us. That's why people come back to read Jungle Red, I believe because we just don't plug our books but make good thoughtful reading.
I love that the cast picture has everyone wearing identical black.
Thank you for sharing this.
R.B.

Hallie, thanks so much for sharing this story about your friendship with Linda, and her tireless efforts to study AIDS and increase the public's awareness of the disease. I was in elementary school when AIDS really hit the public imagination, and there was a lot of initial bias against homosexual men and drug addicts as somehow being responsible for it.

I only remember that attitude sharply changing, at least among my peers, when Pedro on the Real World died from AIDS in the mid-90s, and he was nothing like the stereotypes people believed that AIDS sufferers were. From about middle school onwards, AIDS was part of health class education, and I recall hearing, quite scarily, that during a campus blood drive in my senior year of high school, three anonymous students tested positive for AIDS. Imagine finding out that way.

In any case, thanks again for posting the link to this play. I wish I could see it, but it's the opposite side of the country for me. I'm sure it's going to be fantastic.
R.

"I never intended to become friends with Linda. I have no patience with people who can't keep up. It turned out, neither did Linda."
These three sentences say it all. What a woman!
M.

July 6, 2011
I saw The Normal Heart last week and it was unforgettable. I don't think any other work of theatre has affected me so deeply. I was in tears. What a wonderful tribute to Dr. Laubenstein. Thank you for a chance to learn about the real-life Dr. Emma Brookner.
E.

THE WEDDING

Bruno Albanesi

Come October 22, 2013, Veronica and I will have been married 30 years. Veronica used to work for Linda in her busy practice at NYU, but getting to work and back from College Point was more than an hour long trudge, so Veronica left and Linda went from being a boss to being a good friend.

We saw Linda pretty regularly, meeting either at a restaurant or in her apartment, or at some art gallery where one of Linda's patients was having an exhibit. On one occasion, both Linda and we passed the chance to buy an Andy Warhol at what then seemed a very expensive $5,000.00.

Those of us who knew Linda all know she was undaunted by her challenges. She went about life in Manhattan and elsewhere simply living it with only the slightest of limits. I remember Veronica mentioning the day after a bad snowstorm that Linda showed up at work in her wheelchair, but half the patients cancelled. And in that same spirit, when we told her we were going to get married, she thought nothing of having a reception at her apartment.

We had given Linda the news Veronica was pregnant and that we had decided on a quick and small wedding. Veronica's mother was living in what was then still behind the iron curtain and could not come, so we decided 'friends only, plus my sister and brother-in-law who happened to be in New York at the time. We had arranged for the service at a small chapel in Greenwich and were going to have a reception at a local Greenwich restaurant, but Linda had a better idea: "you guys go get married and I'll host the reception at my apartment." And that she did.

We did as ordered and got married on a beautiful October day in Greenwich. Then with our friends in tow, we headed for 25th Street in Manhattan. We brought the drinks and Linda arranged everything else. Glasses and plates, finger snacks and then a great buffet and a wedding cake. Bill la Rosa, a friend from graduate school, seeing

Linda zooming around her apartment in her wheelchair commented, "You must be very good at Space Invaders."

Linda Laubenstein, M.D.:
Memoir of a Tireless Soldier, Reluctant Hero

Dr. Jeffrey B. Greene

Linda and I both earned our medical degrees at the NYU School of Medicine, she in 1973, and I in 1976. Both of us decided to do our postgraduate training at NYU. Although I am sure I must have noticed her on campus at times, my very first recollection of her at work was during a hematology elective in which she was my preceptor and I was a resident in training. We had been called to the Bellevue Hospital emergency room to see a man in stupor with evidence of widely disseminated cancer. Linda's motorized wheelchair was tough to keep up with as we traversed the expanses of Bellevue hospital to the emergency ward. I can still hear the large rubber tires squeaking on the freshly waxed linoleum tiles floors as she slalomed around objects, some of which were animate, to reach the patient's stretcher. After thoroughly reading the chart and examining the patient, Linda decided a bone marrow exam would be our best first attempt to document what type of malignancy the patient was suffering from. As she prepared her instruments, I asked her if she needed any help. Yes, she replied, please fill out these request forms for the hematology-pathology department. Not the help I was thinking she would need! In the next few minutes I watched with utter astonishment as she removed the left armrest of her wheelchair, moved into position next to the stretcher, and then lifted herself up on the remaining arm rest to begin the procedure. The bone marrow biopsy required screwing in a large bore needle into the posterior iliac crest of the pelvis bone, then tilting the needle in multiple directions to widen the tract, and finally removing the needle which contained a core of bone marrow destined for microscopic examination. Linda needed both hands making her balance tenuous. She never broke a sweat, and didn't hear the confused patient swearing at her. She was totally focused on the task at hand.

In 1981, during my infectious diseases fellowship, I began seeing the very first cases of what was later to be called AIDS at Bellevue Hospital. Linda, now a young hematology-oncology attending, was seeing the first cases of Kaposi's sarcoma, a malignancy associated with AIDS. We worked in parallel spheres but shared our clinical experiences on an almost daily basis. At times we shared patients. As a first year infectious diseases fellow, I was spellbound by the new syndrome, and quickly began to receive calls from physicians around New York City and beyond for advice and counsel on the care of these patients. It was hard to me to balance the excitement of helping to define a brand new disease at such an early stage of my career while remaining cognizant of the physical and emotional needs of those first patients I was treating. Linda had no such conflict and she quickly became my role model. Brilliant and inquisitive she authored many benchmark articles and studies on the treatment of Kaposi's sarcoma. But I never heard her express personal or professional ambition. Rather, her purpose was to become a guidepost for those afflicted with AIDS, helping them optimize their chances of prolonging their lives with dignity and courage. These were the days when the cause of AIDS was still being debated, and years before the availability of antiviral treatments.

In 1984, I hospitalized a young African American gay man with Pneumocystis pneumonia, the "AIDS pneumonia". He wasn't very ill and I had every expectation that he was to survive this first opportunistic infection. Each day I would round on Raymond, I learned more about him as a person. He was a proud man who identified himself by his work. He had a very good job in the fashion industry, his spirits were high, he was a fighter, and couldn't wait to get back to work. Then the unthinkable happened. A pink-slip was delivered by messenger to his hospital room. Suddenly Raymond withdrew, wouldn't speak, frequently was found tearful and he began to decline despite aggressive therapy. He never left the hospital. Raymond was my indelible reminder that within every patient was a person who controlled his own medical destiny despite the drugs and interventions we employed. Linda's early life experiences had long before informed her of the importance of inner strength, self-respect, and the will to live. She and I now shared these revelations and I could now see the basis for her fervent quest for effective treatments.

She knew that providing therapy options was a first step in giving patients the hope they so desperately needed in those early years.

Soon after Raymond died, I passed Linda in the hospital hallway. Still shaken by my failure to cure Raymond's pneumonia, I looked to Linda for solace. She propped herself up in her chair, and looked me squarely in the eyes and said, "His employer's pink slip killed him." In a few minutes it became evident that Linda and I experienced similar instances of desolation and despondence among our patients. We agreed to lunch the following day at the Greek diner across the street from the hospital. During that lunch we conceived of a non-profit organization to advocate for patients in the workplace and to train them for modified positions to allow them to be gainfully employed despite their AIDS diagnosis. We called it MTS (Multitasking Systems). Later we changed the name to Mobilizing Talents and Skills. Our motto was "employment—a treatment that works". I realized early on that Linda had great success in conveying our mission, and was an amazing spokesperson for our nonprofit. She was made president, and convened regular meetings in her apartment on 25th Street, not far from the hospital. During those sessions I experienced first-hand Linda's passion for patient advocacy. She was an inspiration for the group on the board of directors, many of whom had AIDS. I saw Linda develop deep friendships with many of the board members, like soldiers in a front-line foxhole. The intimacy of these relationships was based on a shared mortal threat, mutual respect, and reciprocal energy that elevated the hopes of all involved.

Linda never ceased to amaze me. She was always well-coifed, enjoyed wearing colorful dresses and patent leather shoes and never looked tired or overworked. Linda never discussed her handicap. Her childhood polio had rendered her paraplegic and with diminished breathing capacity. In addition she had asthma and was often seen taking a hit on her handheld inhalers. How she arrived for 7 a.m. rounds every morning was nothing short of miraculous. At one point she successfully petitioned the City of New York to cut ramps into the sidewalks so that daily commute could be safer and shorter. She was a powerhouse.

Linda fought for those who could not fight for themselves. She faced extraordinary resistance amongst her peers in her attempts to develop effective therapies for Kaposi's sarcoma. This tumor occurred almost exclusively in gay men with HIV, but not in other groups similarly infected. This debilitating and debasing disease, with its purple raised lesions, was called by some "the gay cancer". Linda knew that this disease disenfranchised patients, marked them as sick, and worse, announced a person's sexual orientation. Her pioneering work in this area afforded some hope for the large number of patients afflicted with KS. But it placed her at odds with a portion of the oncology community who felt her therapies were overly aggressive. Linda acted as though there was no time to waste in finding effective therapies for KS, and her early results paved the way for established treatment guidelines. She was truly a medical pioneer.

As I got to know Linda over the years, I realized that her iron façade was not as protective as I had originally thought. While on one level she refused to accede to her physical handicaps, she remained challenged to mask the almost supernatural modifications she was forced to make to her life to accommodate them. I recall once, at an MTS fund-raiser at the Americas Club, she was scheduled to give a speech on the ball room floor one story above the lobby. The guests had arrived and her remarks were eagerly anticipated. Unfortunately, the one elevator in the building malfunctioned. Linda began to have a panic attack. How was she going to get upstairs? We agreed to have everyone sequestered in the ballroom while I carried her up the staircase unseen, as others carried her wheelchair. I remember how strangely light this powerhouse of a woman felt in my arms, and how embarrassed Linda was to have to be aided in such a manner. This was my first observation of her emotional vulnerability.

Linda was indeed physically challenged. Once she was hospitalized with pneumonia at Cape Cod Hospital. What should have been a brief illness turned into an ordeal lasting many months. I recall driving up to Cape Cod to see her severely short of breath, thin and very weak. On the way back to New York, I began wondering what her patients would do without her, sure that she would never be able to return to the rigors of medical practice. She amazed me yet again when she returned to the great relief of her afflicted patients.

My wife and children and I would vacation for a week each summer at Linda's house in West Chatham, Cape Cod. Her sense of style was early American, with shaker furnishings, and beautiful gardens and flowerbeds. One year, she asked me to "exercise" her spare electric wheelchair which she left at the house. According to Linda, this was necessary to keep the chair in tip-top shape. I agreed to her request. The day I 'drove' the wheelchair up and down the cul-de-sac I felt an intimacy with Linda that I never experienced before. We had always been close colleagues, but never really developed a social relationship like the ones she had with many of her patients. Navigating her wheelchair along the street put me in a place that allowed me to truly sense her life, her challenges, and her triumphs. I was never as proud of Linda as I was at that moment, and for the first time, I felt she trusted me as a friend.

Linda's death in 1992 at the age of 45 was unthinkable to me, and to so many others. It left a huge void in the lives of so many patients, her family and her colleagues. I regret that she did not live to see the changes in AIDS over the two decades since her death. Antiretroviral therapy, which became available three years after Linda's death, can totally suppress the AIDS virus, and allow the immune system to heal. The dread opportunistic infections we struggled with in those early years, no longer occur in treated patients. Most significantly, Kaposi's sarcoma is almost unseen these days, an eventuality that would have made Linda very happy.

I am constantly reminded of the central role Linda played in the lives of her patients. After her death, I assumed the care of many of her patients. These patients have trouble speaking of her care for them without breaking down in tears of admiration and loss. Their robust health is testimony to the arduous hours she spent fighting the good fight with them. Linda J. Laubenstein was a tireless soldier in the fight against a human plague. And although she would not hear anyone say so, she was a hero to so many that saw her as a penultimate physician, a caring human being, and a valiant proponent for human dignity.

BRIDGE, ANYONE?

Dr. James C. Wernz

I well remember the first time Linda and I went out to dinner together. This was following the holiday party at NYUMC in December of 1976. Linda and I started our hematology fellowship together at NYU the previous July. During the evening with lots of wine we really got to know one another for the first time.

Those who knew Linda well understood her passion for working on NYC to have accessible public transportation for the disabled. It is thanks to her work that the NYC buses now are accessible to the disabled, as are subways. In the early 1990's I lived on the Upper West Side at 97th and West End Avenue and Linda lived in the East 20s. When I suggested to Linda that she come to our apartment for dinner one evening she was very proud to say that she was going to come by bus (with three transfers) rather than having her doorman put her in a taxi with collapsible wheelchair in the trunk and receiving her on my end as we had done for years past. Needless to say, when my doorman announced "Linda here," I told myself—she did it!

Actually Linda and I spent many evenings together over dinner—sometimes out, sometimes with Linda cooking and other times at my apartment. Always there was a nice bottle of wine to mellow the atmosphere and lots of good discussion. This was in the middle of the AIDS epidemic, which added much to the subject matter for our get-togethers. Early on in our friendship we learned that we shared a passion for bridge. Linda became one of the Sunday afternoon regulars for bridge and dinner at my apartment.

Linda was fiercely independent which was underscored by my visit to her family home in Barrington, Rhode Island, just outside of Providence. She planned this while her parents were away showing that she could be the perfect host by herself. This was the weekend of the wedding of one of our NYU oncology nurse specialists in Boston. I had rented a car and picked Linda up at her building that Saturday morning. That weekend not only did we enjoy the wedding festivities (ceremony at Old North Church), but also a side-trip to Newport on a gorgeous day. I still remember Linda out there on the bluff with the wind blowing through her hair.

My Buddy Linda

Margie Vasquez

Linda and I had a relationship on many different levels. We were colleagues, she was my family's physician and of course, most importantly, she was a close friend. Let me start.

Linda was a physician, hematologist, when I worked as an oncology nurse at NYU Medical Center. We started seeing some of the first young male patients diagnosed with Kaposi's sarcoma, a type of cancer associated with a different population. Needless to say we joined forces, I went on to be a part of The AIDS Clinical Trials Unit as a research nurse, Linda had started doing some of her own research, and we collaborated on several projects and from there, started a lifelong friendship.

When my mother was diagnosed with a type of Myeloma, Linda was there with her expertise, determination and compassion. Mom loved her as a daughter.

When my brother was diagnosed with lung cancer, though we consulted with a solid tumor oncologist, it was Linda he trusted, respected and liked. He knew she would always give it to him straight and with compassion. Afterwards they would start talking about gold, which they both enjoyed.

Linda was my friend; how I miss her. We could be on the phone for hours late at night, we frequented the theater, went out to dinner at least once a week, trying out as many ethnic restaurants as we could and of course visited all the museums. We were always scheming on new ways on how to meet men in NYC. Linda had a dry sense of humor, we both loved to laugh and we made a great team.

We had a funny story we called "On the Way to the Wrong Museum". Linda called me and said, "I have two tickets to an exhibit at the Met (Metropolitan Museum of Art), 82nd St and 5th Avenue." It's winter. We trek uptown to the museum. When we get there we decided to check our coats, Linda had a short mink. The coatroom attendant tells us they can't accept fur coats because of the liability.

Anyway, we go back and forth (by this point the museum is going to close in an hour). Linda tells him she won't hold him responsible, finally he calls his supervisor. The supervisor arrives, we express our concern about missing the exhibit, etc. He proposes we put the fur in his locker for safekeeping. I suppose to shut us up. We rushed to the admissions attendant with our tickets; she promptly tells us the exhibit is not at this museum, but at the MOMA. She was right. I suggested we go ahead into the museum anyway, after all we had made such a stink at the coatroom. Linda vetoes the idea, concerned that it's getting too late. We decided to get our coats and leave, but of course we don't want to tell the clerk or supervisor we had the wrong museum.

Linda comes up with the line about her being a physician and she's just been called, there's an emergency, she has to return to the hospital and says it all with a straight face.

We left, coats in hand and with sympathetic comments about life as a physician. As we get outside it's snowing, we decided we deserved the snow for the lies we've told; then promptly traveled back downtown and ordered takeout.

MY DEAR FRIEND LINDA

Eric Wolff

I consider myself privileged to have known Linda Laubenstein and to be able to call her a friend. I got to know her while she was treating a friend and colleague of mine, Gyles Fontaine, with whom I had a performing company back in the 1970s and 1980s. Linda was extraordinarily compassionate and supportive of him until his passing in 1985.

Our performing company's home was our loft in Tribeca where we would rehearse and build our props and sets. We frequently performed there for small audiences as well, showcasing the works that we would perform at the International Experimental Theater Festival each year as well as shows that we could perform in various Off Broadway Theaters that existed in those days in Soho.

This was back in the early days of Tribeca and our elevator was still the same clanky, open caged dinosaur that was first put in the building. The building is a brick and timber building dating from the mid-19th century and the elevator had been added after the building was built but was a relic of the early 20th century at the latest. This was no deterrent to Linda who insisted on coming to the loft to see one of our performances. This required that she brave being carried up the narrow stoop of several steps in her electric wheelchair and riding on the elevator. It took four of us to manage the stoop, which was quite narrow. The ride up the elevator was always an adventure with its greased wooden rails, bare brick shaft walls, and clankety-clank sound. The way you made it go was to pull up or down on the looped chain that hung in the corner of the shaft.

The only concession Linda demanded was that we go out for dinner, rather than eat at the loft, after the show so that none of us who helped with the chair had had anything to drink before she was back on solid ground again!

When my daughter was born in 1991 Linda was ecstatic, delighting in her arrival almost as much as my wife and I did. She was always eager to have us all come by so that she could enjoy Simone's developing personality. Simone took a shine to Linda as well and was happy to sit in her lap and gaze into Linda's dark eyes.

One evening she invited us for a dinner, making sure that we dressed up a bit as she wanted this to be a special occasion. When we arrived she had set the table beautifully and had created a spot for Simone's carrier on the table so she could be at eye level with us all. Living as she did in a chair Linda was very aware of the difference it made to be at eye level rather than below it. She had cooked a beautiful dinner and had arranged the dinner to present Simone with a beautiful antique child's rocking chair. Later, she also presented Simone with a white blanket that she had crocheted. Both of those things remain precious to my daughter who is now about to graduate from college.

Another quintessential memory of Linda for me is the story of her helping me when I developed asthma. I had had a bad cold, one that was going around that year and after the cold was gone I was still wheezing. I thought I had bronchitis and Linda referred me to a pulmonary specialist who was a colleague of hers. He turned out to be out of town so Linda told me to just come over to her place. When I arrived she got out her stethoscope and took a listen to my chest. "You don't have bronchitis," she said, "You have asthma!" She went into her bathroom and emerged with a big handful of pills. There were a number of different medications (Linda had asthma so she was well stocked) and she handed it all to me. "Take these," she said.

"How many? Which ones when?" I asked.

"All of them—now," was the answer.

She then had me sit with a vaporizing inhaler for a dose and I felt much better. I finally had the appointment with the pulmonary specialist and got everything stabilized but I was on steroids for a few weeks. As I was finally getting off them, cutting the dose down every day I had made a plan to have dinner with Linda and my wife at a restaurant in Greenwich Village. While I was working that afternoon I was having all sorts of strange emotions wash over me and I was having crazy thoughts about jumping out of the window and feeling paranoid. I didn't know what to make of it. This was not like anything I had ever experienced.

When I got to dinner Linda was sitting there with Gina. "Hi, Eric, how are you doing?" she asked. I was still feeling rather weird as I sat down.

I told her about what I had been experiencing that afternoon and she just laughed. "That's just the prednisone withdrawal; it makes you 'hormonal'. Now you have some idea of what PMS is all about!"

I'll never forget my dear friend Linda.

ON MEDICAL RESIDENTS

Dr. Richard Ostreicher

Linda had the proverbial heart of gold but she was a tough taskmaster when it came to the training of the internal medicine residents. Medical school and residency were difficult for her due to her physical challenges, and yet she mastered the art of performing physically difficult medical procedures as well as nurturing her humane spirit to genuinely care for the emotional well-being of the people who put their lives in her hands. She would subsequently accept very few excuses from her residents for a poorly done job involving patient care. The resident who didn't do the appropriate sepsis workup when a patient 'spiked' a fever was sure to hear about it within hours of the offense. And the resident who treated her patients disrespectfully would almost certainly be looking to make sure all of his or her body parts where intact and functional after Linda had her "little chat" with the offending young doctor.

The residents were terrified of Linda (well, at least the new recruits or ones of questionable competence). As it happened, Linda's motorized wheelchair made a buzzing sound when she was in full forward throttle, and this was enough to clue the acute listener that Linda was on her way. Sometimes, by the speed of the buzz one could tell if Linda was on the warpath, and residents would duck into closets, around corners, or under desks or counters—anything to escape the wrath of Dr. Laubenstein.

Linda knew all this, of course, and used it to her patient's advantage. She once told me that she would sometimes show up on the hospital ward unexpectedly and 'buzz' around for an hour or so, just to encourage the residents. "There's nothing like generating a little terror to get a job done," she wisely advised.

DOCTOR INSPIRATION FOR NORMAL HEART CHARACTER

Kathi Scrizzi Driscoll
Cape Cod Times

Chatham—Priscilla Laubenstein has the dress ready.

That's the message she emailed to playwright Larry Kramer when he told her that The Normal Heart, his 1985 groundbreaking play about the first days of the AIDS epidemic, was finally getting a turn on Broadway.

The play opened in previews Tuesday and will have its official opening night Wednesday at the John Golden Theatre on West 45th Street. That night, Priscilla Laubenstein will be dressed up to walk the red carpet with her son, Peter, Kramer, and other celebrities to watch actress Ellen Barkin make her Broadway debut playing the character inspired by Priscilla's daughter, Dr. Linda Laubenstein. Barkin will perform with a cast of well-known theater and TV names to re-create the dark days that Linda lived through and made such a mark on.

Kramer says he invited Priscilla because she wanted to see the production, and because of Linda.

"Linda herself would never come and see the play when it was at the (off Broadway) Public Theater (in the '80s), no matter now hard we tried to get her there," Kramer said in an email interview. "Priscilla, quite rightly, is a fervent advocate for her amazing daughter's memory and legacy. Linda will be played here by Ellen Barkin, an amazingly brilliant actress who is just in love with this part and I know will please Priscilla."

This Broadway show is a big event for many who knew Linda: Priscilla and Peter plan to have dinner Tuesday with many of her friends (some of who tried and failed to get tickets to the sold-out opening); Linda's dentist is attending, and other family members have gotten tickets for later in the 96-performance run.

Attending the opening night "is going to be very fun and exciting, but I'm mostly excited for Larry Kramer—that he's getting the recognition he deserves, that Linda was a part of that (play) and that she's getting the recognition she deserves," Priscilla says. "Would that all doctors were like her."

Priscilla and Peter live in the Chatham home that was Linda's getaway and where she died unexpectedly in 1992. The home has the easy access and ramps that Linda needed for the wheelchair she'd been in since age five (because of polio). Many pieces from Linda's art collection—most gifts from patients, including a Mexican-style portrait of her that includes an angel's halo—hang on the walls alongside the Cape art collected by Priscilla (a trustee of the Cape Cod Museum of Art for nine years) and Southwestern pieces belonging to Peter.

Priscilla confirms that Linda never saw Kramer's play and the Dr. Emma Brookner character he modeled after her, his partner's doctor, down to the wheelchair. "She did tell us one day, very casually, 'Larry Kramer wrote a play that I'm in,'" remembers her mother. "She didn't talk about it at all. That's not what she was about."

Priscilla has seen the play a couple of times ("it isn't hard for me"), including with Barbara Bel Geddes and when acclaimed actress Julie Harris, a Chatham neighbor, played Linda in a staged reading at Cape Cod Community College and used Linda's own electric wheelchair onstage.

It was that mid-1990s fundraiser that first prompted Priscilla to contact Kramer, and the two have corresponded occasionally since, mostly by email.

For more than a decade, Barbara Streisand had the film rights to The Normal Heart—with plans to play Linda herself—and Kramer kept Priscilla updated about the fits and starts of a hoped-for movie version. The "having a dress ready" joke between them had been about a Hollywood premier, Kramer says, but then this Broadway opportunity came about after a successful 25th anniversary staged-reading benefit last fall for which Glenn Close played Linda.

Joel Grey directed that reading and Joe Mantello (a Tony Award-winning actor for Angels in America who has become better known as a director of such shows as Wicked) starred as Ned Weeks, who is based on Kramer. Both Grey and Mantello are onboard for Broadway, along with theater and TV star John Benjamin Hickey (The Big C),

Patrick Breen (Broadway's Next Fall), and TV stars Jim Parsons (The Big Bang Theory) and Lee Pace (Pushing Daisies) in their Broadway debuts.

The play—advertised on its website as "Larry Kramer's masterwork of love, rage and pride"—is the story of the early days of AIDS, of "a city in denial ... that unfolds like a real-life political thriller—as a tight-knit group of friends refuses to let doctors, politicians and the press bury the truth of an unspoken epidemic behind a wall of silence."

Kramer, whose writing has made him a finalist for both an Oscar and Pulitzer Prize, co-founded the Gay Men's Health Crisis—which describes itself now as the world's first and leading provider of HIV-AIDS prevention, care and advocacy—and he founded the AIDS Coalition to Unleash Power (ACT UP), a protest organization that was key in changing public policy and perceptions about people living with AIDS and HIV.

Thinking back to the era that Kramer wrote about in The Normal Heart, Priscilla called it "a very scary time." She says Linda was "a pioneer, because no other doctors would see patients with AIDS. So she stepped up to the plate." Linda co-wrote the first paper related to the AIDS epidemic and co-organized the first medical conference on the disease.

Priscilla says Kramer and Linda spoke often, and her vision of the future of AIDS affected him: "She realized what this ... pandemic was going to be. She could see the future. She understood that it was not a gay men's disease; it was everyone's disease and it was going to be worldwide." Because of this, Priscilla says, Linda talked for hours with Kramer and supported his activism to get the word out and make people pay attention.

Priscilla remembers her daughter as a very smart scientist and a compassionate and understanding doctor who was always calling her patients, even when she was in Chatham, and even if they were overseas. Linda also tried to call public attention to AIDS and helped to found Multitasking, a nonprofit organization that retrained AIDS patients, many of whom had been fired from other jobs.

"She is incredibly important in the history of AIDS, a genuine pioneer and a real fighter for what she believed," Kramer was quoted as saying at the time of Linda's death. In the recent email interview, he said: "Dr. Linda Laubenstein was a great, great person, a supremely gifted physician who was devoted to her patients, all of whom adored her. At one point, she was taking care of more AIDS patients than any doctor in the entire world, which took a great toll on her health but did not stop her for a second. She invented or developed the original combination of chemotherapies that are still used to this day. She was beyond brilliant and beyond courageous. I have never known anyone like her and I hope that my play does her the honor she deserves."

With Streisand no longer owning the movie rights to this story, Priscilla has heard and read rumors of other plans to make a movie version of The Normal Heart (it's listed on the Internet Movie Database as due to be released in 2012). Priscilla understands that celebrities sell tickets, but wonders who might play her daughter as so many actresses who have played Linda—who died at age 45, a decade after she started working with AIDS patients—are really too old for the part. (Barkin, for example is 58; Close is 63.)

Priscilla has high hopes that the coming weeks will change that kind of casting.

"After this play goes to Broadway, they aren't going to need celebrities to finally get the movie version made," she says.

In Memoriam

Dr. Jeffrey Greene

We have come together today to pay our respects to Linda Laubenstein who was so unexpectedly taken from us last Saturday. Many of us sitting here share the same remembrances of this wonderful woman, who brightened the lives of everyone she touched. I had the privilege of knowing Linda as a mentor, a colleague and a friend.

My first recollections of Linda were taken from afar. I was a senior student in medical school, and she was a resident in training at Bellevue Hospital in New York. I have images of her tending to sick patients in the oppressive and oft times foreboding surroundings of a municipal hospital emergency room. I was very timid and impressionable at that time and I never mustered up the courage to speak with Linda then. But her movements and manner were decisive and she appeared as a strong and confident leader.

Later in my training as resident I worked closely with Linda for the first time, during a hematology elective. Linda was a brilliant diagnostician who thrilled at the complexities of her field. Her energies seemed limitless, and I was amazed at the respect this young physician was shown from her more senior colleagues. Linda was a marvelous teacher who knew when to challenge, and when to reward her students. I never felt unimportant around her, nor did I ever dare cut corners.

During my infectious disease fellowship, in 1980, Linda was an attending [physician] who had just begun her private practice. Her brilliance as a diagnostician led her to detect the very first cases of what was later to be known as AIDS. She immediately recognized that those isolated cases were the first glimpse into a horrifying new epidemic that was to change the world forever. It was only fitting that Linda was the first American physician to be mentioned in Randy Shilt's chronicle of the AIDS epidemic, And the Band Played On. She was the driving force behind the earliest research efforts at the NYU

Medical Center. Linda became my mentor, and my role model. She instilled in me the love of clinical investigation, and the importance of intellectual integrity. At the same time, her patients were never allowed to feel like research subjects. I learned from Linda the importance of human dignity as a weapon against disease.

As the epidemic marched on, so did Linda. She rose to the needs of patients with Kaposi's sarcoma, a rare AIDS related tumor, and pioneered the earliest effective treatments. Linda was recognized worldwide as the expert in this field, and she participated in conferences, organized symposia, planned research protocols, and wrote scores of papers on the subject. Her tireless efforts were truly remarkable and for me, inspirational. In her private practice, Linda did not limit herself to the area of hematology/oncology. Rather, she became a consummate AIDS physician, one who learned how to treat all aspects of this complex illness. Linda would never relegate the care of her patients to a panel of consultants. She was always at the helm, and the patients loved her for it. In her strength, they found the fortitude to battle against the unspeakable odds of AIDS.

By 1982, I entered private practice and modeled my career after Linda's. I was advised by many of my fellow physicians not to become known as an AIDS doctor. I must admit that I had some ambivalence about the grueling nature of an AIDS practice. Linda's perceptions about this were clear. A doctor must respond to a patient's needs, regardless of the personal sacrifices this entailed. She pointed me in the direction of sensitivity and logic and thankfully, I followed her lead. At that wonderful moment, and for the first time, Linda and I became colleagues. We were frontline soldiers fighting side by side in a battle against an incalculable enemy. I cannot imagine a closer professional relationship, nor one in which I could ever respect another more.

Over the next several years, Linda and I shared many patients. She always seemed to know them better than I. I don't mean their case histories. I mean them, their lives, their loved ones, their stories. She made house calls, she on occasion socialized with them, and she knew them as people, not as cases. Linda could never be judgmental although she was often opinionated, and the doctor-patient relationships she nurtured were very special. We saw platoons of people die before us, and the legacies they left behind bonded Linda and me closer than ever. Our professional affiliation transformed slowly into a friendship that I will always treasure.

In 1986 I saw a patient who was fired from his job the moment a diagnosis of AIDS was made. The pink-slip, not the disease, killed my patient. As I commiserated with Linda her eyes widened, and I could see the wheels of her mind begin to turn. At that moment, Multitasking Systems of NY, Inc. was conceived. This nonprofit organization was created to provide a work place for persons with AIDS. Linda believed that work was therapeutic in the fight against chronic illness. Over the years I had the privilege of seeing Linda direct MTS as an officer. Her expertise in the boardroom, at fundraisers, on television interview, and in motivating those of us involved in the project rivaled her abilities as a physician. The very existence of MTS today, years later, is directly attributable to her unwavering efforts on behalf of all HIV infected people. I am very proud to have worked with Linda at MTS, which stands as a monument to Linda's sense of commitment and her fortitude.

As our friendship grew, I saw Linda in many different ways. She was cultured, enjoying the theater, fine dining, and the arts. During our board meetings at her apartment in Manhattan I always saw a different book at her bed stand. Linda's pet cats were a continual source of enjoyment for her. Cape Cod was always a special place for Linda, and she took great pride in her home, her garden, and her neighborhood. Linda would usually return from the Cape tanned and invigorated, and tell me about the divine new restaurant she tried, or the crafts fair she browsed through. Linda loved Shaker furniture, and she was an accomplished needle-worker. Christmas time brought handmade sweaters for my youngsters. Those of us who stayed at her house in the Cape were greeted by explicit instructions and household rules taped to the refrigerator door. She loved her home, and loved to share it with her friends. My wife Miriam and my two children will always share fond memories of our Cape Cod vacations.

In early 1990, Linda became ill while visiting her home in Cape Cod. Her illness was prolonged and life threatening. I visited her in the ICU of Cape Cod Hospital and for the very first time, saw my friend as weakened and helpless. Despite her brush with death, she instructed me from her iron lung to go back to NY with positive news. Her own fears aside, she wanted her patients to believe that she would be back for them. During the long drive home, I could not imagine Linda ever returning to work as an AIDS practitioner. But, as we all know, her spirit prevailed and she was back to full time practice until last week.

Those who did not know Linda well had trouble ignoring her wheelchair, and her 'handicap'. Linda though, in my eyes, may have been physically challenged, but she was never handicapped. Her accomplishments were limitless, testimony to her inner strength and brilliance. Linda hid from any situation that attempted to portray her as handicapped. She resisted her character in Larry Kramer's The Normal Heart. In another instance, during a fundraiser for MTS, the elevator from the mezzanine was turned off and Linda had to be carried down a flight of stairs. Sensitive to her embarrassment, I bid everyone farewell and cleared the premises before carrying her to the main level. No, she would not be seen as handicapped, because in life, handicapped she was not!

Linda J. Laubenstein achieved a level of greatness in her brief years that eludes many a lifetime. She has added focus and meaning to my life and I am forever in her debt. My heartfelt sympathy goes out to Priscilla and George, and Peter. I pray we can all find solitude in Linda's loving memories.

IN MEMORIAM

Dr. Edward L. Amorosi

I first met Linda Jane almost 20 years ago when she was a medical student on an elective in Hematology. On a few afternoons she worked with me seeing patients in the office. To say the least, it was a little cramped in the original faculty practice offices—especially with a second person in a motorized chair. Nevertheless, we enjoyed working together and it was clear and obvious that Linda was someone special.

She was intelligent, interesting, witty, well organized and courageous beyond belief. Who can forget the sight of Linda on her way home, after a long hard day, in the dark of night—both winter and summer—alone in a chair—and fail to appreciate the courage displayed by this woman every day of her life?

In 1980, Linda, Bob Silber, Simon Karpatkin, Henriette Lackner and I moved into new quarters in the present Faculty Practice Offices. Later Drs. Raphael, Hymes, Smith and Goldenberg would join us. Our respect for Linda knew no bounds. She had excellent judgment, great ingenuity and a woman's intuition, which were an unmatched combination in caring for patients with complicated medical illnesses. She never expected special consideration and carried her full share of the clinical and teaching responsibilities of the group—just as she had during her arduous residency and fellowship years.

Her interests and activities were not confined to medicine. She dressed beautifully. She was a real New Yorker—having always seen the latest Broadway plays or musicals; having always been to the latest hit movie or the newest chic restaurant. She always had tickets to special exhibits at the Met or Museum of Modern Art and regularly attended her favorite—the New York Flower Show. She had a garden on her terrace in the city and had just showed me and the nurses in Coop the latest photographs of her garden in Chatham the week before she went to the Cape for what proved to be the last time. It was a beautiful English country garden with a large variety of flowers—

and Linda had the most obscure names of these plants at her fingertips. I promised to show her photos of my more modest gardening efforts when she returned from the Cape. Unfortunately, we never shared that pleasure.

Everyone is aware of her major contributions to the clinical description and definition of AIDS and to the care of patients with this disease. I remember her excitedly telling me about the first few young men with Kaposi's sarcoma whom she, Ken Hymes, Jeff Greene and Alvin Friedman-Kien had seen and recognized as a new clinical entity. She became famous and was almost overwhelmed by the number of patients clamoring for attention. While she was recuperating from surgery a few summers ago, I visited her on her back porch in Chatham and asked if she was up to coming back to such a difficult task. She was uncertain then but within a few weeks was back on the job again with her customary energy and efficiency and was still at it two days before she left us.

As our number of patients increased, the new quarters in Coop Care had again become cramped and she was anxiously looking forward to our contemplated move to new offices in the Skirball building. She looked forward to this not only because it would be more commodious for all of us and especially for her but primarily because it would provide greater comfort for her patients. She was always very concerned about not only her patients' medical problems but their emotional and mental well-being as well.

Two days before she left for vacation we had a meeting regarding the new office space. Linda was having asthmatic problems and I told her to take good care of herself at the Cape because we all needed her. She indicated that there was no need for concern, that she would always do her share and in fact was on call the weekend before she left for the Cape.

It would be difficult to find a more dedicated, valiant, and talented physician. She contributed so much to her friends, her students, the house staff, her patients and colleagues. I am sure that she had achieved her eternal reward for a job well done in too short a period of time. We will remember her forever and miss her very much.

IN MEMORIAM

Flora S. Davidson, Associate Dean, Barnard College

Others here are more qualified to speak of Linda's extraordinary contributions to medicine and her patients. I am here to evoke Linda in her years as a student at Barnard and as a loyal alumna. I was privileged to be Linda's classmate at Barnard, and during the past few weeks I have been gathering memories, my own and those of others with whom we shared our undergraduate years. The words that came first—from everyone—were motivation, strength and courage. Linda thrived on being independent and self-sufficient. In those who knew her, bouts of self-pity or self-doubt were short lived. If she could manage it, how could we complain? And not only could she manage, but she did so with warmth and an engaging sense of humor. We all remember that dazzling smile—a smile that lit up her whole face.

Like others of us, Linda chose to come to Barnard for its challenging liberal arts education, its concern for women's issues, its affiliation with Columbia University, and the opportunities of New York City. But unlike most of us, Linda also chose Barnard for what it did not have—a sprawling spacious campus with rolling hills and wide-open spaces. How lucky for Barnard! For once, our modest campus was an asset!

For Linda, Barnard meant self- sufficiency—a compact four square blocks, with a same-level tunnel system connecting all buildings- residential as well as academic. She sought and she found physical accessibility in a supportive community. And how quickly she learned to get around in the city, in the days before public buses had wheelchair lifts, becoming expert at getting into taxicabs.

Linda loved her years at Barnard and spoke proudly and often of them. She majored in Biology and took the heavy science program one expects of a pre-med. But she was entranced by American and European art, music, the Modern Novel, and Shakespeare. She credited Barnard with honing her eclectic and wide-ranging interests—in the arts, music, reading, travel, and yes, even fine dining. That must have been one of her off-campus activities!

She maintained the friendships she forged in college all her life (with people like Pam Gallagher, Hallie Ephron, Pat Hunter, and Sandy Biller, who are here today). She served as Vice-President of our class and helped to organize our 15th Reunion. She made regular contributions to the College and helped raise funds from our classmates by helping out with telethons. She took every opportunity she could to give something back, and even arranged to leave a bequest to the College.

When Barnard formally established the Office for Disabled Students in 1977, Linda pitched in to get the word out to others. She is featured as a working physician in one of its brochures and quoted as saying, "Ten years ago with no help it was a minimal problem for a disabled student to attend Barnard. With a little help and some of the positive attitude that Barnard possesses, I think that Barnard is a place with a tremendous amount to offer. And there aren't many places like it around. … Even with physical accessibility now mandated by law, it takes a lot more than obeying the law to create surroundings that minimize problems for disabled students."

That Linda went on to do the groundbreaking work she did when she left Barnard is clearly a credit to her own extraordinary talent and dedication. She was an exemplary role model before that term was fashionable.

Barnard is as proud of Linda as she was of Barnard.

PATIENTS' LETTERS

ROSEMARIE

Dear Dr. Laubenstein,

Please [I] apologize for not having written to you earlier. I kept thinking of writing all through the year but was too sad to find the right words to thank you for all you have done for Rene.

Rene had the best treatment at the Lucerne Hospital but he kept saying how much he missed you, not only as his doctor, but also as a good friend who had accompanied him through the painful but always hopeful years of his illness with AIDS. He had been hoping to come back to N.Y. until his last day—and if it was just for a few days— especially to see you and to talk to you about his experience with Swiss doctors, his hopes and fears and his sadness about the loss of Nathan.

I am grateful that Rene could pass away so peacefully with Ursula and myself holding his hands. His last word was "flowers" and that gives me hope that everything was alright for him at the silent moment of his passing away.

Dear Dr. Laubenstein—in my thoughts you belong to Rene's last three years of his life and I shall never forget the strong support you have given him during this period. I hope that life is good to you and that you will always find a new strength to deal with this terrible illness.

With my best wishes for 1991 and kindest regards.

Sincerely yours,

Rosemarie

BILL

Dear Mr. and Mrs. Laubenstein,

Forgive me for such delay in communicating to you my feelings of your loss, our loss. I've started to write a card several times, but somehow it didn't seem like enough. I felt I needed to say more than the space in the card will allow. Even though there isn't enough space or proper words to even begin an attempt to describe all I'd like to say about Linda.

You need not be reminded I'm sure of the person she was, and will always be in our lives. When we lose someone that is a part of our lives, there aren't words to properly convey what one goes through. Linda and I nursed my partner through over 200 days of continuous hospitalization. He passed away this past December 6th. We almost made 13 years. He was the biggest and most important part of my life.

I can't begin to comprehend what you as parents must feel. For me, Linda was my doctor since the mid 80's. It didn't take long till she was my best friend. She gave me such a sense of security with my own HIV status that will never be equaled. I still don't have a doctor even though I've been through seven. I suppose I should stop comparing, knowing there will never be an equal.

We were from the very beginning 'friendly' rivals of our flowers and gardens. Each spring/summer we'd always bring and compare pictures of our plants. My specialty is peonies and lilies, with about 50 peony plants and dozens and dozens of iris. This past spring I had nearly 800 blooms on the iris. She loved them. When I took the album into the office she asked to keep it so she could show some others, obviously that made me very proud.

One more week and I would have divided one of my iris beds intending to share them with Linda. I was planning on coming to the Cape and plant them for her. Every time I see an iris now I'll think of her, bringing to the surface many memories.

I'm sure you saw the Blue Granny Square and Ripple afghan she had in her bedroom. I made it for her a while ago. When she opened it, the expression on her face was one I had never seen before. It was one of such little girl excitement. Without doubt one of my proudest memories.

I trust you still have it? I would only hope and would want you to use it for as long as you'd like, look at it as a reminder of what she meant to her patients, meant to her. She took it out in the waiting room and proclaimed it was made by me, if anyone could top it she'd see them next. I'm sure you heard Linda speak of Mary Gocke. She's a nutritionist that was working on a drug program called Marinol. I've grown very close to Mary. Mary and I were both disappointed to learn you weren't going to be able to attend the Memorial Service at the University, but we understand. Keeping in line with my feelings for Linda, and the relationship Linda and Mary shared, I have a request. Reluctantly I ask for fear I'm out of line. However, should you ever decide to part with the afghan, may I request you give it to Mary? I feel this would please Linda very much. I know Mary would cherish it and take pride in the history it holds. Thank you.

Again, may I say you're in my thoughts and prayers? God bless you with courage for understanding you loss.

Bill

LINDA'S MILESTONES

1947: Born May 21, Boston, MA, parents, George and Priscilla Laubenstein.

1952: November Contracted polio and hospitalized in a negative pressure ventilator (iron lung) at an infectious disease facility.

1953: Released to home in Barrington, RI in February 1953.

1956: Attended Nayatt Elementary School.

1958: September, first operation for spinal fusion; encased in full body cast for one year.

1958: In the sixth grade Linda was connected to class via an intercom system, which allowed her to participate in all class activities from home. Classmates would bring homework assignments to her twice a week, which she would complete from her bed. One outstanding assignment was an autobiography of her life.

1960: Graduated Junior High at West Barrington Junior High.

1963: Awarded a Merit Scholarship by Everest and Jennings, Co.

1964: Graduated Barrington High School.

1964: Entered Barnard College, New York City, as a pre-med student.

1968: Graduated Barnard College.

1972: Graduated New York University School of Medicine.

1972: Interned at University Medical Center, New York.

1974: Two year residency in Hematology; Bellevue Hospital, Veterans Administration Hospital, NYC and University Hospital, NYUMC.

1977: Began clinical practice with Hematology Group, NYUMC.

1978: Instructor of Clinical Medicine at NYU School of Medicine.

1981: Published "Thrombotic Thrombocytopenic Purpura after Heterosexual Transmission of Human Immunodeficiency Virus (HIV)" in The Lancet

1983: Assistant Professor of Clinical Medicine, at NYU School of Medicine.

1984: Co-sponsored first international symposium on "The Epidemic of Kaposi's Sarcoma and Opportunistic Infections" edited by Linda J. Laubenstein, M.D.

1986: Incorporated Multitasking, Inc. with Dr. Jeffrey Greene. Multitasking, Inc. was a nonprofit organization established to employ people with AIDS and offered office services, word processing and desktop publishing services to businesses.

1992: Died, August 15, as a result of a massive coronary occlusion.

Posthumously elected a Fellow of the American College of Physicians.

Linda Laubenstein, M.D. Award established by the New York Medical Society for outstanding clinicians in the field of AIDS.

CURRICULUM VITAE

Linda J. Laubenstein, M.D.
530 First Avenue
New York, NY 10016

DATE OF BIRTH: May 21, 1947

EDUCATION

1969   A.B., Barnard College
1973   M.D., New York University School of Medicine

POSTGRADUATE TRAINING

1978   Fellowship, Division of Hematology
            New York University Medical Center (NYUMC

1973-76   Internship and Residency, Straight Medicine,
            NYUMC (Bellevue Hospital)

ACADEMIC APPOINTMENTS

1983   Assistant Professor of Clinical Medicine, NYUMC

1978-1983   Instructor of Clinical Medicine, NYUMC

1974-1978   Teaching Assistant, NYUMC

BOARD CERTIFICATION

1978   Subspecialty Certification in Hematology

1977   American Board of Internal Medicine

SOCIETY MEMBERSHIP

            American College of Physicians
            American Society of Hematology
            New York County Medical Society

1. Friedman-Kein AE, Laubenstein LJ, Marmer M et al:
   Kaposi's Sarcoma and Pneumocystis Pneumonia Among
   Homosexual Men- New York and California. MMWR 1981;
   80: 305-8.
2. Hymes KB, Greene JB, Marcus A, William DC, Cheung T,
   Prose NS, Ballard H, Laubenstein LJ: Kaposi's Sarcoma in
   Homosexual Men- A Report of Eight Cases. Lancet 1981 Sep
   19; 2(8247): 598-600.
3. Marmor M, Kriedman-Kein AE, Laubenstein LJ et al; Risk
   Factors for Kaposi's Sarcoma in Homosexual Men. Lancet
   1982 May 15; (8281): 1083-7.
4. Krigel R, Ostreicher R, LaFleur F, Laubenstein LJ, Zang E,
   Wernz J, Friedman-Kein AE. Epidemic Kaposi's Sarcoma
   (EKS): Identification of a Subset of Patient's With a Good
   Prognosis. Abstract, ASCO Annual Meeting, Houston, Texas,
   May 19-21, 1982.
5. Friedman-Kein AE, Laubenstein LJ, Rubsenstein P et al:
   Disseminated Kaposi's Sarcoma in Homosexual Men. Ann
   Intern Med 1982 Jun; 96(6): 693-700.
6. McCauley DI, Naidich DP, Leitman BS, Reede DL,
   Laubenstein LJ: Radiographic Patterns of Opportunistic Lung
   Infections and Kaposi's Sarcoma in Homosexual Men. AJR
   1982 Oct; 139(4): 653-8.
7. Rose HS, Balthazar EJ, Megibow AJ, Horowitz L,
   Laubenstein LJ: Alimentary Tract Involvement in Kaposi's
   Sarcoma: Radiographic and Endoscopic Findings in 25
   Homosexual Men. AJR 1982 Oct; 139(4): 661-6.
8. Krigel RL, Laubenstein LJ, Muggia FM: Kaposi's Sarcoma:
   A New Staging Classification. Cancer Treat Rep 1983 Jun;
   67(6): 531-4.
9. Friedman-Kein AE, Laubenstein LJ (eds.): AIDS: Epidemic
   Kaposi's Sarcoma and Opportunistic Infections. Masson
   Publishers, New York 1983.
10. Marmor M, Friedman-Kein AE, Zolla-Pazner S, Stahl RE,
    Rubinstein P, Laubenstein LJ, William DC, Klein RJ,
    Spigland I: Kaposi's Sarcoma in Homosexual Men: A
    Seroepidemiologic Case-Control Study. Ann Intern Med 1984
    Jun: 100(6): 809-15.

11. Cooper JS, Fried PR, <u>Laubenstein LJ</u>: Initial Observations of the Effect of Radiotherapy on "Epidemic" Kaposi's Sarcoma. JAMA 1984 Aug 17; 252(7): 934-5.
12. Ziegler JL, Beckstead JA, Levine Am, Lukes RJ et al: Non-Hodgkin's Lymphoma in Homosexual Men with Lymphadenopathy or AIDS. Clinical Features in 90 Patients Six Institutions. N Engl J Med 1984 Aug 30; 311(9): 565-70.
13. <u>Laubenstein LJ</u>, Krigel R, Odajnyk C et al: Treatment of Epidemic Kaposi's Sarcoma with Etoposide or a Combination of Doxorubicin, Bleomycin and Vinblastine. J Clin Oncol 1984 Oct; 2(10): 1115-20.
14. Krigel RL, Odajynk CM, <u>Laubenstein LJ</u>, Ostreicher R, Wernz J, Vilcek J, Rubinstein P, Friedman-Kein AE: Therapeutic Trial of Gamma Interferon in Patients with Epidemic Kaposi's Sarcoma. J Biol Response Mod 1984 Aug; 4(4): 358-64.
15. Pennington JE, Groopman JE, Small GJ, <u>Laubenstein LJ</u>, Finberg, R: Effect of Intravenous Recombinant Gamma-Interferon on the Respiratory Burst of Blood Monocytes from Patients with AIDS. J Infect Dis 1986 Mar; 153(3): 609-12.
16. <u>Laubenstein LJ</u>, Raphael B, Chachoua A, Scholes J, Mousalen J, Metrokin C: Clinical Manifestations of B-Cell Hyperplasia in Response to HTLV-III/LAV Infection. Abstract, Int. Conf. Acquired Immunodeficiency Syndrome (AIDS), Paris, France, June 23-25, 1986.
17. Berger CL, Friedman-Kein AE, DiFranco M, Rehle T, Ostreicher R, Knobler R, Donofrio S, <u>Laubenstein LJ</u>, Edelson RL: Tumor-Associated Antigen is Expressed on Lymphocytes from Patients with Acquired Immunodeficiency Syndrome. J Invest Dermatol 1986 Aug; 87(2): 280-3.
18. Wernz JW, <u>Laubenstein LJ</u>, Hymes K, Walsh C, Muggia F: Chemotherapy and Assesment of Response in Epidemic Kaposi's Sarcoma with Bleomycin/Velban. Abstract, ASCO Annual Meeting, Los Angeles, CA, 1986.
19. <u>Laubenstein LJ</u>, Kamelhar DL, Garay SM, Greene JB, Poiesz B: Lymphoid Interstitial Pneumonia (LIP) in Adult AIDS. Abstract, Conf.., AIDS, Paris, France, 1986.
20. Chachoua A, Dieterich D, Krasinski, K, Greene J, <u>Laubenstein LJ</u>, Wernz J, Buhles W, Koretz S: 9-(1,3-Dihydroxy-2-propoxymethyl) guanine (Ganciclovir) in theTreatment of Cytomegalovirus Gastrointestinal Disease With the Acquired

Immune Deficiency Syndrome. Ann Intern Med 1987 Aug; 107(2): 133-7.

21. Leaf A, Laubenstein LJ, Raphael B, Hochster M, Karpatkin S: Thrombotic Thomocytopenic Purpura Associated with HIV Infection. Ann Intern Med 1988 Aug; 109(3): 194-7.

22. Rivers JK, Laubenstein LJ, Postel Am, Valentine F, Knowles Acute Monocytic Leukemia in an HIV Seropositive Man. Submitted for Publication.

My Family

Linda Laubenstein, age 10

There are four in my family, dad, mom, Peter and myself. There is also a cat named Lola who thinks she is the boss.

Dad is always busy. He likes to build and draw. Many of the things he has designed are for me. Dad and I are interested in watching and identifying birds. He has built several birdhouses for me. Dad has always said he was not a lover of cats. However, who's out in the middle of storms, or climbing trees to get the cat? Dad.

Dad was born in Cleveland, Ohio. There he lived until he was in high school when he moved to Hingham, Massachusetts. Dad has always liked music. While in high school he organized a band in which he played the saxophone. After graduating from Bowdoin College, he went to Annapolis and in due time became commanding officer of a minesweeper in Japan. In 1945 he married Priscilla Martin who is now my mother.

Mom was born in Boston, Massachusetts, where she lived until she was four. Then she moved to Milton, Massachusetts. After graduating from Connecticut College she worked at the Massachusetts Institute of Technology. There she did research work on uranium ore for the Manhattan Project. Another research project Mom worked on was treating penicillin to increase its yield.

Mom likes to cook. At Christmas we have fun helping her make cookies. She also enjoys having company whether it is hers or ours. After dinner is game time when we all enjoy playing cards or some other type of game. Both Mom and Dad like to garden. Dad prefers vegetables, while Mom likes flowers.

My brother Peter was born August 1, 1951. He can best be described as mischievous. One time near Christmas he found a jar of red ink which was supposedly out of reach. The jar opened and spilled all over Peter and the chair. If you care to look, it is still there. His worst day was when he decided to make coffee and threw the grounds all over the kitchen. Later that morning he dumped a jar of tomato juice into the white wash. For days we slept on pink sheets. Furthermore that afternoon he sampled a can of Bab-O.

We have been led to believe that Peter is running for mayor of Barrington for it's anybody's guess where he is after school. Although he doesn't get into quite so much trouble now, he manages to keep things lively.

This story wouldn't be complete unless I included Lola. She is our cat who thinks she's a person. There is nothing she likes better than to sit on the dining room table or climb the drapes.

One morning she wanted to go out. She couldn't awaken Dad so she went half way across the room, took a running leap, and landed on Dad. Needless to say she went out. Every day she goes to school with me. Sometimes she gets up on the table and attacks me.

Although she's the world's biggest pest, I wouldn't trade her for anything. I enjoy my family.

MY FRIENDS

Linda Laubenstein, age 10

I have many friends. I think I'm very lucky to have so many because
without friends life would be pretty dull.

My first real friend's name was Gail O'Connor. Although she is a
little older than I am, we got along very well, although we did have
arguments. One thing that we always wanted to do was catch a bird.
We believed that to catch one you had to put salt on his tail. We
would take saltshakers and go out in the field and try to get one.
Unfortunately we never succeeded. Another thing we liked to do was
to play dolls. We washed their clothes quite often in the birdbath. I
don't think they got very clean but it was fun. After a while Gail had
to move. Every once in a while I see her because she now lives in
Boston.

For the next few years I didn't really have many friends because I
wasn't in school. When I did go back to school, I became very good
friends with Nancy Smith. We played together almost every day. One
day when we were playing a game my brother, Peter, drank some
shellac and turpentine. Mom took him and tried to make him throw up
but couldn't. I went down to Nancy's house while Mom took Peter to
the hospital. On the way down we had to go through some tar. We
didn't think to wipe it off the wheelchair and we got it all over her
mother's new rug. It all ended all right because Peter was sick on the
way to the hospital. Nancy now lives in Pennsylvania. We write to
each other occasionally. I hope that I will see her again some day.

Another friend of mine is Liz Taft. She lives in Florida now but
she used to live in Connecticut. Her mother and father are friends of
ours. She has come to visit us twice. When she came she flew by
herself and we went to meet her at the airport. We had lots of fun
when she was here. Every day that it was nice we went swimming and
had a lot of fun. I greatly enjoyed having her visit.

Of all my friends, I like Karen Wells the best. We play together a
good deal. At school she has helped me in different ways, even

though she is in a different room. Both Karen and I like to play with dolls. We have made lots of clothes for them. When I was in the hospital she came up to see me. We had to sneak her in because children have to be fourteen to visit and she is not quite eleven. Whenever she comes over we have a good time. In the summer when she goes to camp I feel lost. If she ever moved, I don't know what I'd do.

Although I have many other friends, too, these are my best friends.

MY PETS

Linda Laubenstein, age 10

We have had many pets including one dog, five cats, a parakeet and a number of fish.

My first pet was a rust colored cocker spaniel. His name was Rusty. I don't remember him very well because I was only three when we had him. One day my friend was teasing him and he bit her so we had to give him away.

The next pet was a yellow cat named Hocus Pocus or Hocus for short. After we had had her for a while she got pretty badly chewed up by a dog. At that time I was in the hospital so we had the vet try to save her. She was in the hospital a long time. When she did come home we nicknamed her "the gold-plated cat". One day when we were at the beach she disappeared and we never saw her again.

Our next cat's name was Sandy. She was a pretty yellow and white tiger cat. Sandy was the best natured cat. She would let Peter, my brother, drag her around or let me dress her in doll clothes. Unfortunately she was run over and killed.

Our next cat, Posy, looked just like the others. I guess I liked yellow cats. After we had her for a couple of weeks she was killed by a boxer dog. Since then the dog has been put away because he "graduated" from cats to little girls.

While we had Posy, I got a parakeet for Christmas. It was a pretty bird but it was very stupid. He would just as soon "bite your hand off as look at it". One day when he was out of his cage the front door was open and he flew away. Personally I think that he had some help finding the door from Mom.

Smoky was our next cat. He was black and white. We had only had him a few days when he came down with distemper and died.

We now have another cat named Lola. About two years ago she had four darling kittens. Their names were: Ginger, the prettiest, who was orange and fluffy; Butterscotch, my favorite, who was white with yellow spots; Salt and Pepper, who was black and white; and Sugar, the best natured, who was yellow. One day Sugar disappeared when we were going to give her away. We hunted all over and finally found her in a neighbor's car. To this day we don't know how she got there. About two months afterwards Sugar came back while her owners were away. Karen Wells and I decided to dress her in doll clothes. After we did that we got a doll's bottle and fed her with it. Any other cat would have been "as mad as a wet hen" but Sugar just lay there.

Of all the pets I've ever had, Lola, the cat we have now, is my favorite. There's only one trouble with her, she thinks she's a person.

SCHOOL DAYS

Linda Laubenstein, age 11

When I was five, I started kindergarten. I went to Nayatt School. My teacher was Mrs. Gardner. In November, just after Halloween, I had polio. I was in the hospital about four months, and that was kindergarten.

When it came time to start first grade I was still unable to go to school. I had a teacher come to my house. Her name was Miss Shay. She came three times a week. On nice days we would sometimes have school outside. We had a lot of fun and I learned a good deal but I would have rather been in school.

Again in second grade I had a tutor. This time I had Mrs. Grace for a teacher. I liked her very much.

In third grade I went to school. I was very excited the first day. I had Mrs. Pierce for a teacher. I will never forget the time I had my first dictation test. Everybody else had had some English the year before, but I hadn't. I don't think I had anything right on the whole paper. That was a rude awakening! Another experience I remember was when I was playing with my ruler and I put it under my chin. All of a sudden it broke in two. Everyone looked around. I was never so embarrassed in my life!

In fourth grade my teacher was Miss Redfern. I was out of school most of the year because of three operations. At the hospital I was in, they had school for the children. There were seven girls in my class, ranging from second to sixth grade. My teacher was Mrs. Isebelle. I didn't like her too much. One of the girls had cerebral palsy. She did all her work on the typewriter with her head. She wore something like a football helmet with a stick on it. She was very smart. When I was home from the hospital I had the intercom. It was more difficult that year than it is this year. Toward the end of the year I went back to school.

For fifth grade I had Mrs. Morse. She was a good teacher and I learned considerably. During the first half of the year I was the librarian. I liked that job a lot. The second half I was vice president of the class. I didn't like that job at all. There was hardly anything to do besides sitting next to the president at meetings. Another thing I remember is that for a couple of weeks my pencil disappeared every night. Some of the girls would tease and say that I ate them. It got to be quite embarrassing asking the teacher for a new one everyday. One thing that I hated was "Maxon Cards". We had to do four and it seemed as if I did a hundred before I got four perfect ones. If I had to pick my favorite teacher, it would be hard. I have liked all of them but I think my first grade teacher, Miss Shay, was my favorite one.

HOBBIES

Linda Laubenstein, age 11

I think my hobby is one of the most interesting there is. It is watching and identifying birds. Birds are very pretty, even though some people think they are pests.

I first became interested in birds when I was about seven. To start with we had one bird feeder, now we have three. One of them is right next to my window where I can watch them anytime. I have seen many kinds including sparrows, gold finches, purple finches, chickadees and evening grosbeaks. At the other feeder we have; starlings, sparrows, flichers [sic], blue jays and others. Today we saw the first sign of spring: redwing blackbirds. In with the redwings we saw two boat-tailed grackles. These birds are very large, about seventeen inches long. This is the first time I have ever seen one.

The prettiest birds I have ever seen is an indigo bunting. They are a very nice shade of blue. I saw it about three years ago in April. I happened to be home because I was sick. I'm very glad I was.

Another pretty bird we have are evening grosbeaks. I first saw them January 20, 1958. This year on the twenty-first of January we saw them again and have had them ever since.

In the summer time we have birds like robins, goldfinches, brown thrashers, bandit warblers, catbirds, and yellow warblers.

Of all the birds my favorites are the bandit warbler, chickadee and field sparrow. I like the bandit warbler because he is so cute. It's named bandit warbler because of a black mark across its eyes. The chickadee is always very busy. One time he hollowed out a stump in the yard for his nest. It looked so funny to see him sit in the tree spitting sawdust all over the place. I like the field sparrow because he is so friendly. He likes to sit on my bird feeder and stares in at me.

This winter I have especially enjoyed watching the birds because I am in bed all day. I am a member of the Massachusetts and Rhodes Island Audubon Societies.

VACATION DAYS

Linda Laubenstein, age 11

Vacation days are always fun. I have had many exciting ones. The following ones are my favorite.

One of my favorite vacations was my trip to New York. When I first had polio my grandmother promised me that when I was up and around again she would take me to New York.

During spring vacation when I was in second grade we went. On the afternoon we flew down we saw a play called "Pajama Game". It was a musical and it had a lot of good songs. The next day we went to see the Gary Moore show. After the show he came down and talked to me. Then we went back to our hotel to meet a couple of friends for lunch. That afternoon we went to Radio City Music Hall to see the "Rockettes". That night we had dinner with my uncle Bill. He had a surprise for me. It was tickets to see the ballet. He also took us up on top of the R.C.A. Building. It was quite a thrill to look down and see the cars and people. They looked just like toys.

On Friday we saw the circus. I had my picture taken with Emmit [sic] Kelly, the famous clown. It was the first time I remember seeing the circus. The next morning we went shopping and I got some clothes. That afternoon we went to the ballet. We saw "Peter and the Wolf", "Billy the Kid", and "Helen of Troy". Of all the things we did I liked this best.

Right after the ballet we went to the airport to come home. There wasn't room on the seven o'clock flight so we had to wait around until eleven o'clock at night to get a plane. If I had to pick my favorite vacation, I think this would be it.

Another vacation I enjoyed was a trip to Franconia, New Hampshire. It took almost a whole day. We stayed at a place called Lovett's. It was very nice. Across the road there was a dammed up brook where we swam. The water was freezing cold, but we had fun.

One day we went up to Cannon Mountain. Mom decided that she didn't want to go. I loved going up in the tramcar but Peter cried all the way. When we got to the top he said he wasn't going down in the car and started to run away. Dad had to leave me and go chase after him.

Another day we went to the top of Mt. Washington. It was a beautiful day when we started but by the time we reached the top it was cold and cloudy so we didn't see too much.

On another day we went to an Arts and Craft Shop. I bought a miniature wooden village. Every year at Christmas we set it up. One afternoon we went to an auction. Mom bid on one thing but didn't buy it. All too soon we had to go home. Yes, vacation days are fun.

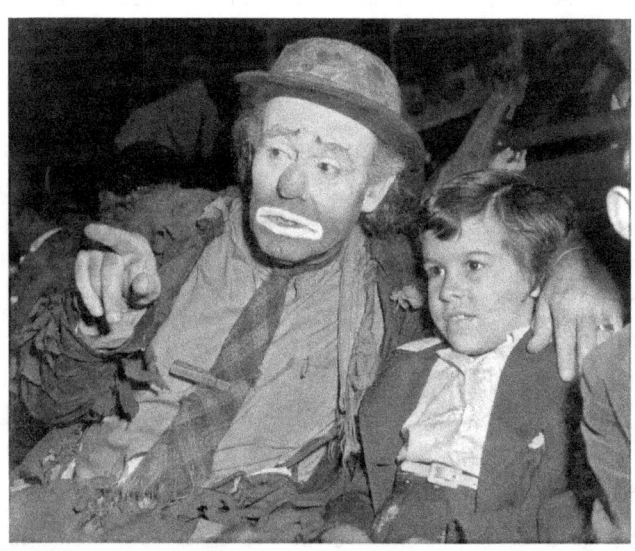

Sixth Grade

Linda Laubenstein, age 11

This year is my last year at Nayatt School. My teacher is Mrs. Walkden. For science Mr. Steel comes in on Monday and Friday. He has had us make two science projects. My first one was a model steam engine with its parts labeled and an explanation of how it works. The second project was a water filter. Our classroom is the largest in the school. It has a stove, refrigerator, electric stove and planting area. One wall is lined with closets containing many well-used ditto papers. Along the windowsill are many boxes filled with different kinds of plants.

At the beginning of the year the class had lessons with Miss Demery at the public library. For about eight weeks I was in the hospital having a spinal fusion. Since I have been home in a cast I have gone to school over the intercom. At Christmas time we had a party for my whole class at my house. It was a little crowded but we had a lot of fun.

Every other week on Wednesday, Mr. Hawkes comes and teaches us about nature. Before each lesson we have a question period. Different people bring in things dealing with nature that they have found and ask questions about them. Every year the P.T.A. gives a graduation program for the sixth grades. This year Mr. Steel gave a talk about science and the weather. Our class wrote the words for a "farewell" song which the three sixth grades sang together. After the "graduation" Mrs. Walkden and Diane, Betsy, Kathy, Lisa, and Judy came over for a little while to visit.

This year is my last at Nayatt School. Next year I will be in a new school but I will never forget my years at Nayatt, the teachers there, or the friends I have made there.

www.ingramcontent.com/pod-product-compliance
Lightning Source LLC
Chambersburg PA
CBHW051729170526
45167CB00002B/858